Parkinson's Treatment:
The 10 Secrets to a Happier Life

English Edition

By **Michael S. Okun, M.D.**

ISBN: 1481854992
ISBN-13: 9781481854993

Table of Contents:

Author's Prologue:

THE RECENT FORECASTING ESTIMATES FOR Parkinson's disease are staggering. If accurate, the numbers suggest an urgent need to wake up and recognize that we are on the cusp of an emerging pandemic. It is frightening to consider that in the world's most populous nations, the number of Parkinson's sufferers will double to almost 30 million by the year 2030. These escalating statistics may seem unbelievable, but they are real, and they are fueled by a continuously aging population. Age is the unavoidable and undeniable risk factor underpinning the development of Parkinson's disease. As life expectancy increases, so too do the number afflicted. Put another way, if everyone lives to be 100, we will be forced to deal with Parkinson's disease, and it will be a worldwide crisis.

In travelling the world as the National Medical Director for the National Parkinson Foundation, I have met tens of thousands of Parkinson's disease sufferers, family members, and friends. One of the most common questions on their minds is "what can I do to make my life and the lives around me better?" I wrote this book to help quench that thirst that is shared by Parkinson's patients and families worldwide. It is in that spirit that through our network of former fellows and colleagues we have translated this book into as many languages as possible in order to get the word out about the secrets to hope and a happier life with Parkinson's disease.

Introduction:

THE FOUR SIMPLE WORDS "YOU have Parkinson's disease" will pierce the heart and drain the dreams of 50,000 people world-wide each year. Once the shock of the diagnosis subsides, four new words will dominate the thoughts of each sufferer: "Is there a cure?" Today, the answer is no. Each new sufferer will, following diagnosis, unconsciously step onto a crowded, shuffling and often shaky road.

Lu Xun, a prominent 19th and 20th century Chinese writer who reflected on mortality and humankind penned, "Hope cannot be said to exist, nor can it be said not to exist. It is just like roads across the earth. For actually the earth had no roads to begin with, but when many men pass one way, a road is made.[1]" Thus, we can conclude that each successive generation of Parkinson's sufferers have added to this long road. Some bystanders will occasionally extend themselves to reach out to those who pass on the Parkinson's road. Others, free of disease, will for various reasons choose to journey with the Parkinson's travelers. The "others" will provide the hope, the light, and the science critical to fuel any chance of reaching the road's end.

Listening to thousands of Parkinson's disease sufferers, I am deeply inspired. Their rich history and experiences provide all the motivation necessary to press on toward a cure. This is why the stories yet to be discovered will be as important as those we have already heard. This book will piece together and distill the best and the most critical of these stories that are helping map a road to a happier and more meaningful life for the Parkinson's disease patient. Throughout the book we will consider the major "hits" and "misses" in the symptomatic treatment of the disease. Understanding the rationale, the science, and the empiricism behind each will greatly enhance the sufferer's, the caregiver's, and the family's knowledge base. Connecting the dots and dispelling some of the mystery of Parkinson's disease will reveal the hidden path toward hope and happiness.

The first time I see a patient and family unit, I am greeted by a Curious George style squint and a long sigh. The scenario vividly reminds me of a trip I took early in my career to New York and to the Michael J. Fox Foundation for Parkinson's disease research. I was one of Fox's first grant recipients, and when I sat down to dinner, a man from UCLA whispered to his friend at the table, "Is that Okun? I thought he would be much older." Frequently I overhear a spouse or wife uttering a similar phrase. Some people might guess that I would be offended by those words; however, the honest truth is that I relish hearing them, for they mark the beginning of my journey with a treasured patient and an important family unit. They mark what I hope will become the spark to ignite the light of hope that will help to guide to a destination that includes a happier and more meaningful life. Over the years, I have grown with each of my patients, and their journey is my journey.

One thing I acquired from my father was the ability to sense and appreciate critical moments in life. Steve Jobs once said to his team, "Everyone here has the sense that right now is one of those moments when we are influencing the future." Similarly, I appreciate that when I see a patient for the first time, it is my interview. I am applying for a position as "guide" on a journey that will aid in defining many lives. I will be privy to intimate details and family dynamics, and I will be trusted as a confidant and high-level cabinet advisor. Soon everyone in the examination room will have all of my contact information, my emails, my voicemails, and my web addresses. I am acutely aware that my words matter.

I remind myself of Steinbeck's words when I start any journey. "A journey is like marriage. The certain way to be wrong is to think you control it.[2]" No matter how much you plan, how much you save, how careful you are, how much you deserve, you still may end up in my office with a diagnosis of Parkinson's disease. I believe that it is possible to alter the natural course of a journey, and to avoid the many pitfalls that can quickly escalate into a healthcare nightmare.

I constantly find myself asking a core philosophical question about embedding hope in patient-centric care. Is it possible to offer realistic optimism, positivism, and hope, all without offering a quick-fix cure? I believe it is possible. I believe it all comes down to developing your core values and growing your faith. If you develop your core, you will be working with the seed that can grow hope. Mahatma Gandhi taught us that "Faith is not something to grasp, it is a state to grow into.[3]"

That moment when I say "You have Parkinson's disease" is a critical moment. From then forward it will become our shared mission to prevent those two words (Parkinson's disease) from defining a person or defining a family. We must educate the sufferers that people are defined by core values and not by diseases.

I have experienced the marvelous privilege of traveling all over the world and lecturing to patients and families who have been touched by Parkinson's disease. I have been struck and also emotionally moved by the stories, the tragedy, and the courage of those who wake up each day to tackle a new challenge or a new disability. I have since 2006 had the great honor of answering more than 10,000 questions on the National Parkinson Foundation (NPF) Ask the Doctor free international web forum. When I received the call to take over the forum and to sign on as the NPF National Medical Director, I was not prepared for how this experience would change me. The patients and families I have met on my journey have shaped my understanding of chronic neurological diseases in a profound and deeply spiritual way.

The most humbling experience of my life has been the time I have spent with patients suffering from Parkinson's and chronic neurological diseases and with their families. I use the word humbling because time after time, in person, and also on the web forum, we have uncovered simple and addressable issues that have changed people's lives. For some sufferers it has meant walking again, for others it has restored their voices, and for many it has resulted in the lifting of a depression, anxiety and desperation cloud that has obscured their dreams and robbed them of potential unrealized happiness. I have learned while journeying with each of these brave individuals. Together they have helped me to realize listening is critical. Also, they have taught me to never assume a sufferer or family member is aware of the "secrets" that may lead to hope and to a happier life. We must share those secrets.

Though most of the issues facing a Parkinson's and chronic neurological disease patient seem obvious to the many experts in the field, I have become convinced that the majority of patients and families remain unaware of a few simple secrets. These secrets, if revealed, can change their lives. These secrets, if completely embraced, can offer millions of people worldwide hope, better lives, and a more meaningful existence.

The purpose of this book is to share with everyone touched by Parkinson's and chronic neurological diseases the 10 secrets to hope and to a happier life. When I was just beginning to pen the book, I was having dinner with the television commentator Mort Kondracke. He has spent 37 years as a respected journalist and a key contributor to important political think-tanks such as the Beltway Boys, the McLaughlin Report, and Roll Call. Mort's wife was taken care of by my mentors and colleagues at NIH and Emory University. Mort has become one of the most outspoken and important individuals in organizing and advocating for more research and for better care in Parkinson's disease. Ironically, his wife Milly was discovered to have a chronic neurological disease that masqueraded like but wasn't actually Parkinson's disease. Mort convinced me that sharing even small secrets can extend beyond Parkinson's disease and that the secrets of care should be crafted to reach all those suffering with chronic neurological dysfunctions. I have tried my best to follow his advice.

In each chapter of this book I will reveal an important secret and will explain the insight, the rationale, the empiricism, and the science behind it. Additionally, in each chapter I will try to reveal a little more about myself and a lot more about the patients who gifted the secrets. These patients planted the seed of faith. They learned to grow hope, and they discovered the core values necessary to achieve happiness despite chronic disease.

My overall goal for this book is simple. Share the secrets and make them available to everyone, worldwide, who has been touched and may be touched by Parkinson's disease. I am fortunate to have participated in the training of Parkinson's disease doctors and interdisciplinary faculty who now work on nearly every continent. Every day they provide exemplary patient-centric care, and they kindle the hope for this generation and the next. Without hesitation, each of them answered my call to translate this book into their native tongue and to make it available to as many people possible. They are my heroes.

The prevalence estimates for Parkinson's disease are staggering. The numbers suggest an urgent need to wake up and deal with the Parkinson's and chronic neurological disease reality before a worldwide crisis emerges. It is scary to consider that in the world's most populous nations, the number of Parkinson's sufferers will double to almost 30 million by 2030[4]. Because the most important risk factor for development of Parkinson's disease has been identified as age, if everyone lives to be 100, we will all be facing this as a potential large-scale reality.

The aim of this book is to inspire faith, plant the seed of hope, help patients to discover their core values, and use the "secrets" to improve lives. Every patient and every family member touched by Parkinson's and by chronic neurological disease can find and kindle hope. Hope leads to happiness, and happiness will lead to a meaningful life.

CHAPTER 1

Know the Signs

"I look for a sign. Where to go next. You never know when you'll get one. Even the most faithless among us are waiting to be proven wrong."

— Jillian Lauren, Pretty: A Novel

"**D**ADDY JUST ISN'T ACTING RIGHT." "Daddy is shaking." "Daddy isn't picking up his feet." "The bank won't accept daddy's signature." These are some of the common refrains that usually punctuate my initial contact with a family. Though I miss receiving standard handwritten letters, the new generation of technology has empowered families to communicate faster, and more importantly it has set up the possibility for a more engaging and productive doctor-patient relationship.

I teach our young doctors in training that they have a powerful tool that can enhance a doctor-patient and doctor-family relationship—a smartphone. Swift and confident electronic responses can diffuse tense situations and set the appropriate tone for future interactions. The first contact and first response can be critical in achieving a true patient-centric feeling of empathy. There is no replacement for engendering a feeling of true empathy.

Quick validation and decisive action are critical when dealing with patients and families who face tough neurological illnesses. By the time patients or families reach a doctor, one or more of these factors have taken hold: deep-seeded concern, frustration, and anxiety. In the beginning, the best thing a doctor can do is to be highly responsive by immediately scheduling an appointment and by reassuring patients and families there are answers to their questions.

At the University of Florida's Center for Movement Disorders and Neurorestoration, our philosophy is that the service must be impeccable, and every member of the team, including the schedulers, check-in staff, and nurses, must embrace the vision of a truly patient-centric experience. We have found that not only does this approach benefit the patient, it makes us better doctors and builds a better interdisciplinary team. Maya Angelou said, "I've learned that people will forget what you said, people will forget what you did, but people will never forget how you made them feel."

The First Encounter

Several hours to several days later, a medium-sized, focused, and very worried family will predictably present themselves for review. Many times they arrive following an overnight flight or long drive. Painfully, I remember a similar feeling and a similar journey with my dad. Almost every minute of that trip is indelibly marked in my memory, all the while cultivating a strong empathy for others who are suffering.

These worried patients and families will no doubt play back their own initial doctor consult many times in their heads—awake and asleep. In many instances it may be associated with post-traumatic stress as well as vivid dreams.

As doctors, our job is to convince these families that they are at the beginning of a journey and not at the end. The hope started for many of them with a single written plea for help. The existence of that hope must be kindled and ultimately cultivated into a flame that will guide them on their journey.

Part of the buildup of anxiety stems from a family's internal dialogue. It usually considers several relatively common brain diseases as the "contenders" for what is wrong with dad. Suspicion usually circles around four main conditions: Alzheimer's, Lou Gehrig's, strokes/brain tumors, and Parkinson's. Recently I asked a sample of families in the clinic, ranging from main street America to well-known CEO's, if they saw any difference between these four maladies prior to a Parkinson's disease diagnosis. The answer was no. They considered these four diseases to be equally bad—and not just bad, very bad. The common word they used was "devastating."

The good news is that these four conditions are not all the same, which should be a source of great hope. In order to differentiate them you must "know the signs." This is the first secret.

Development of the Doctor-Mentor and Mentor-Educator

One important secret in disease management is learning to not only be a doctor but a doctor-mentor and mentor-educator[5]. This is a concept I learned from Tony Dungy, a successful football coach but an even more successful mentor-educator. The word doctor derives from the Latin word meaning to teach, so as doctors we should earn our keep. We should not forget our roles as "coaches" to our patients.

I have found that there is great value in reviewing the differences between diagnoses, especially in cases where a diagnosis of Parkinson's disease seems to devastate a family member or sufferer. Too many people underestimate the value of teaching and often forget that there are many opportunities for "teaching moments." John F. Kennedy urged America to: "Let us think of education as the means of developing our greatest abilities, because in each of us there is a private hope and dream which, fulfilled, can be translated into benefit for everyone and greater strength of the nation."

Parkinson's is Not Alzheimer's

Since the majority of people worldwide believe that Parkinson's disease is a form of Alzheimer's, this is a good indication that we in the medical community have not done enough to clear up this misconception, and I find this troubling. It does not matter whether I am lecturing in Sioux Falls, S.D., Buenos Aries, London, Istanbul, Bejing, Tokyo or many other patient and research venues. The misconception about Parkinson's being as bad as Alzheimer's exists everywhere.

A deeper look may provide some insight into the misconception. Both diseases are degenerative brain problems. Both result in the death of brain cells. Both transform general appearances, including facial expressions. Both have a visible and serious impact on the family and society. Both result in the loss of billions in wages and in running up healthcare expenditures for all tax-paying citizens. Finally, both diseases have the potential to cloud memories and transform personalities. I cannot count how many times I have heard from a spouse: "He is just not the same man I married." Given the similarities, it is understandable that people equate Parkinson's and Alzheimer's and even use common adjectives when describing both—devastating, untreatable, and indignant.

Therefore given the background of the public's perception, it is critical to make sure, as doctor-mentors and mentor-educators, that people understand Parkinson's disease is not Alzheimer's disease. Teaching families to recognize and appreciate the differences will empower them and will kindle hopeful thoughts.

It is critical that those who are suffering as well as their families understand that Parkinson's is not Alzheimer's. A direct comparison between the two will reveal obvious and important contrasts in clinical symptoms and disease course. The analysis of critical brain tissue has unlocked the understanding of the differences between neurodegenerative diseases. The brain allows us an opportunity to clearly show that all three conditions (Alzheimer's, Lou Gehrig's, and stroke/brain tumors) commonly confused with Parkinson's disease are different entities.

Alzheimer's disease is a neurodegenerative disorder, so cells die in the brain. The condition can lead to symptoms such as memory loss, confusion, hallucinations, behavioral disorders, and difficulty thinking. A small percentage of patients with Alzheimer's will manifest similar features to those encountered in Parkinson's: stiffness, slowness, tremor, gait problems. When there is any symptom overlap, it may result in an identity crisis for patients and also families. In the rare instances when doctors are having trouble differentiating the two entities, a neurologist with expertise in movement disorders can distinguish them or order a high-power scan called a positron emission tomography scan for definitive differentiation.

Common motor symptoms of Parkinson's disease include:

- Tremor (not present in 20 percent of cases)

- Stiffness (rigidity)

- Slowness (bradykinesia)

- Gait and balance issues

- Small handwriting (micrographia)

Common non-motor symptoms of Parkinson's disease include:

- Depression, anxiety, and mood disorders

- Apathy

- Psychosis (illusions and hallucinations)

- Cognitive dysfunction (thinking problems)

- Autonomic dysfunction (low blood pressure when standing, gastrointestinal problems, constipation, sweating, urinary issues, sexual dysfunction)

- Sleep disturbances

Over the years, some of my favorite patients have had Alzheimer's disease. Jim, a tall, skinny university professor, was one of them. We shared a love of history, political science, and the humanities, and we would reminisce about common books we had read. We would talk about the past, and I would help Jim when he couldn't find the right words to finish his sentences. Gradually, however, Jim lost all of his memories for recent interactions, and sometimes he even got lost trying to navigate to his appointment. If I walked out of Jim's room and immediately walked back in, it was like someone jokingly hit the restart button on his hard drive. The previous interaction seemed to just evaporate. This is the scenario that plays out repeatedly in the course of a single day for more than five million families in the United States, and my experience with Jim has given me an important glimpse into the frustration and heartache that plagues families battling Alzheimer's. Spouses and families have decades of stored memories and shared histories, and in a stroke of what may feel like cosmic sarcasm, they too find themselves lost. They are filled with the symptoms of caregiver strain and left asking questions such as: "Is this dad?" or "Is this the man I married?" This stereotypical pattern of memory loss, word-finding problems, and disorientation does not commonly occur in Parkinson's disease patients and is a critical difference between the two diseases. This is an important distinction. As doctor-mentors we need to be sure our patients and families understand the critical difference between the two diseases.

Alzheimer's disease is associated with the brain deposition of a protein referred to as Tau. If you apply a brown Tau stain to brain tissue, it will reveal the plaques and tangles that help to pathologically distinguish and define Alzheimer's.

Parkinson's disease, in clear contrast, is associated with deposition of a different protein, referred to by scientists and clinicians as alpha-synuclein. In 1912, Frederick Lewy, a pathologist who was born in Berlin but later practiced in the United States, stumbled upon the discovery of peculiar brain accumulations. These accumulations have been referred to as protein deposits, and they have been proven to be strongly associated with Parkinson's disease. The deposits Lewy observed have been widely thought to be linked to the underlying issues resulting in the disease itself. The collections of abnormal proteins were named in his honor and are now called Lewy Bodies[6, 7].

It has always been strange to me how the medical field races to a big discovery and then names a terrible disease after the "discoverer." Naming treatments makes more sense to me, so I think I will pass if someone tries to attach my name to a disease or disease protein.

The point of telling Frederick Lewy's story is to emphasize that we have an obligation to teach patients and families about the underpinnings of degenerative diseases and the differences between them. A deeper understanding and familiarity of these issues will help to foster hope.

Another level of evidence that Parkinson's and Alzheimer's are different lies in the brain regions they attack. Most people can be taught to understand the importance of different brain regions in dictating what symptoms a disease may reveal. After Albert Einstein died, his brain was closely examined and dissected in an attempt to appreciate differences and to help explain his underlying genius. It was widely reported that the areas important for spatial memory and for mathematics were larger than expected, and this may have accounted for at least some of his superhuman abilities. In Einstein's brain the changes in specific regions yielded "features" or enhancements[8]. Diseases, however, usually cripple one or more brain regions. The crippling effect is the primary reason a neurologist can examine eye movements, facial features, mental status, strength, and reflexes and then proceed to localize a deficit to one or more very specific brain regions. In Alzheimer's, the primary region and the first affected is the one essential for memory, whereas in Parkinson's disease, the primary or initial region traces to areas important for smell, sleep and digestive functioning. Understanding symptoms (knowing the signs) and knowing that each symptom may trace to specific brain regions will help patients and families appreciate why certain diseases exhibit specific patterns and result in specific symptoms.

As Parkinson's disease unfolds, abnormal proteins spread from lower brainstem regions to higher ones, or regions that are referred to as cortical regions. In the process of spreading, the proteins disrupt many motor and non-motor brain circuits and lead to important and often visible manifestations.

Some scientists, such as Nobel Prize winner Stanley Prusiner, believe that the spread of Parkinson's throughout the brain mimics infective agents. Prusiner is most famous for his discovery of proteins in the brain called prions. These proteins can, in pathological states, lead to a rapidly progressive dementia referred to as mad cow or Creutzfeldt-Jacob syndrome. (Again, ironically named after the two neuroscientists who originally described it.) For years no one believed Stan. His colleagues, friends, and the National Institutes of Health all turned their back on him, and many laughed at his notions of disease and disease spread. Prusiner, however, was proven correct about prion proteins. Additionally, he has recently drawn attention to the notion that proteins can migrate and act like infections in the brain. This possibility provides an intriguing explanation for how disease spreads within the brain tissue[9].

Is it plausible that the brain proteins that cause Parkinson's disease are really an infection-like manifestation? As it turns out, long before Prusiner began talking about his theory many scientists interested in the field appreciated that protein processing had already been considered to underpin this idea. Interestingly, several of these scientists described a unique reaction. When healthy dopamine cells were transplanted into human Parkinson's-diseased brains, they were found to be sick with the Parkinson's proteins. Though it is true that the bad proteins spread throughout the brain, it is not believed that Parkinson's disease is caused by an infection. The exact reasons for the behavior of these bad proteins and also their function remain a mystery.

After the initial months and years of degeneration, Lewy Bodies begin to creep beyond the deep brain regions and insidiously leak into areas involved in both motor (tremor, stiffness, slowness) and non-motor function (depression, anxiety, apathy, sexual dysfunction, memory, thinking). Patients suffering from neurological disorders and their families need to appreciate that in brain real estate, there is nothing more important than "location, location, location." Location dictates symptoms.

In contrast to Parkinson's disease, Alzheimer's patients have early onset cognitive and memory symptoms. In Parkinson's disease, cognitive symptoms are milder and usually present many years into the future. Scientists believe the reason for the late presentation in Parkinson's is that it takes time for the degeneration to spread from the deep brain circuits to the "higher" areas involved in cognition and behavior[10, 11, 12]. This George Bernard Shaw quote, "Everything happens to everybody sooner or later if there is time enough," unfortunately captures how many of the changes in Parkinson's and Alzheimer's occur through the normal aging process.

Current symptomatic treatments for Alzheimer's disease include the use of a multi/interdisciplinary team, cholinesterase inhibitors (which stimulate a chemical called acetylcholine, known to improve memory), memantine (a chemical that stimulates glutamate and is important for learning and thinking), as well as the use of behavioral training and education for the affected patients and families. The available drugs and approaches in Alzheimer's disease in most cases have only been mildly beneficial, and the effects on memory usually wane quickly.

On the other hand, the treatment for Parkinson's is usually more robust. The replacement of a chemical called dopamine can result in an "awakening." Additionally, several other pharmacological strategies have enabled the modern Parkinson's disease patient to live many full and meaningful years before any motor or non-motor disability is revealed. These years offer the hope for a chance at achieving substance and meaning in one's life.

Differentiating Parkinson's from ALS

While ALS (amyotrophic lateral sclerosis or Lou Gehrig's disease) is frequently confused with Parkinson's, its differences can be easily distinguished once patients and families have the right information. Lou Gehrig's disease results from the loss of nerve cells in a layer of the spinal cord called the anterior horn. In this disease the cells are lost, and they cannot adequately communicate with the body's muscles. This condition can lead to muscle twitching, wasting, and weakness. Muscles in the throat and chest can become involved and affect speech, swallowing, and breathing. About 10 percent of cases are genetic, and most cases have a very short disease duration from diagnosis to death (two to five years).

Many Americans believe that a typical course for ALS is like that seen in Stephen Hawking the famous English theoretical physicist. However, in practice, patients need to be aware that Hawking is an outlier, and that ALS, unlike Parkinson's, is a rapidly progressive and notably different degenerative disease. ALS has its own unique protein deposits, which is why they are referred to as Lewy-body like[13].

Lou Gehrig was known as "The Iron Horse" of baseball until 1995 when Cal Ripken Jr. broke his record. Gehrig played in the most consecutive games (2130) in baseball history. His streak was broken by his disease when he benched himself because he felt the power had exited his arms and legs. In 1939, during Lou Gehrig Appreciation Day, he proclaimed in a famous speech he was the "luckiest man on the face of the earth." Gehrig died in 1941. It is important for patients to understand that Parkinson's is vastly different from the rapidly progressing muscle-wasting disease that benched baseball's Iron Horse.

Differentiating Parkinson's Disease from a Stroke or Brain Tumor

Sometimes in the clinic, Parkinson's disease patients can present with hypochondriasis and anxiety. For many years it was assumed that these issues were "stress," but we now know that they may be commonly associated with part of the actual degenerative disease process. The fear of a stroke or brain tumor can interfere with care and negatively impact outcomes. For an overly anxious patient and on rare occasions, I may order a brain scan for reassurance.

Thankfully, the differences between Parkinson's disease and a stroke or a brain tumor are relatively easy to explain. One of the first symptoms of Parkinson's may be an arm that does not swing when walking. It is not uncommon for this to be the initial clue that prompts a phone call, an email, or an in person consultation. Often these patients have had a brain MRI that reveals no stroke and no tumor, which may leave their doctors perplexed.

The former president of Princeton University and the 28th president of the United States collapsed in 1919 after a bitter fight about joining the League of Nations with Henry Cabot Lodge. Woodrow Wilson won the Nobel Peace Prize. In 1919, Wilson was in the process of reshaping post-WWI empires into peaceful coalitions. However, 1919 was not a good year for him. This would be the year he would largely disappear from the public eye due to the devastating effects of a stroke that resulted in right-sided weakness, partial blindness, and uneven thinking. His disability was hidden from the public for the majority of the next five years, and though he partially recovered, much of what had been lost was never regained[14].

Strokes are focal areas of brain tissue that die when not nourished with oxygen. The biggest and most important difference to appreciate between a stroke and Parkinson's disease is that a stroke is usually non-progressive, meaning the deficits do not get worse. Strokes also typically attack a specific brain region. Finally, unlike strokes, Parkinson's does not lead to weakness or what has been referred to as hemiplegia.

Similarly, a brain tumor attacks a specific region, but unlike a stroke, the disability usually evolves and worsens over the course of the disease. The evolution may be comparable to Parkinson's, but there are many glaring differences between brain tumors and Parkinson's disease.

Brain tumors are collections of abnormal cells that continue to divide and expand until they form disruptive globs within the skull. These globs can have associated brain swelling and can press on or disrupt normal brain function. In simple terms, the regions of brain affected by a brain tumor usually directly predict the symptoms encountered. A good neurologist should be able to determine the regions affected based on talking to a patient and family and then performing a complete bedside examination.

Brain Tumors

In 1937, President Franklin Roosevelt ordered his staff to immediately determine the location of the most famous neurosurgeon in the world, Harvey Cushing. It was a national emergency. The American icon and musical hero George Gershwin was lying in a California hospital bed with severe brain swelling, and Roosevelt was briefed that Gershwin may soon die. When the staff found world famous neurosurgeon Harvey Cushing, who was then retired, he recommended Walter Dandy, who happened to be vacationing on a yacht in Chesapeake Bay. Unable to call Dandy, the Coast Guard retrieved him from his boat; however, it was too late for Gershwin. Dr. Eugene Ziskind at Cedars Lebanon Hospital in Los Angeles would perform emergency surgery, but Gershwin would not survive.

Gershwin had, over the preceding year, been developing headaches, and he complained of "smelling trash." Not unexpectedly with those symptoms, he ended up in a psychiatric hospital. His apathy and behavior confused his doctors and led to a delay in his diagnosis. The problem Gershwin was facing was an uncontrollably growing tumor, and the tumor was pressing on smell centers in the brain as well as causing seizures, leading to peculiar behaviors. The swelling would eventually lead to weakness, uneven pupils, and death[15, 16].

It is important for Parkinson's disease patients to be aware of stories such as Gershwin's and to appreciate that the pattern of symptoms and the rapidity of the disease course, though progressive, is not consistent with Parkinson's disease. Other famous sufferers including Lou Gehrig with ALS and President Woodrow Wilson with a stroke help to illustrate the distinctions between Parkinson's.

Brain tumors have actually helped us to better understand Parkinson's disease. In 1893, Paul Blocq and Georges Marinesco described a case of a tumor in the region of the brain that is home to dopamine, also called the substantia nigra. The two doctors described a patient who had a tremor and appeared to be affected with Parkinson's. The tumor pressed on a vital region of the brain and eventually resulted in Parkinsonian symptoms but not actually Parkinson's disease[17].

These tumors are very rare. When they do occur, the symptoms are only on one side of the body, and patients almost always develop true weakness or paresis. Weakness and paralysis are not symptoms of Parkinson's disease. Parkinson's is actually a slow degeneration of motor and non-motor circuits that involves both sides of the brain. Additionally, it encompasses numerous brain regions and brain circuits.

The History of Parkinson's Disease

Parkinson's disease, erroneously termed paralysis agitans, was previously described in the Indian medical system of Ayurveda (called Kampavata) and also by Galen (A.D. 175) who referred to it as the "shaking palsy." Perhaps the most famous reference can be found hidden in a work of Shakespeare who wrote in Henry VI: "Why dost thou quiver, man?" The character in the story responded by stating "the palsy and not the fear provokes me." The use of the term Parkinson's disease was largely credited to the highly influential 19th century French neurologist Jean-Martin Charcot, although it should be noted that many people prior to Parkinson himself described the disease. James Parkinson (1755-1824), a Londoner and son of an apothecary, is credited with the eponym for his 1817 essay on the shaking palsy. His descriptions included six cases, only three of which were actually examined. (Two were met on the street and one simply observed.) One of the most curious and inspiring points about James Parkinson is that he was not a neurologist but an insightful and observant family doctor[18].

Parkinson's Disease: The Basics

There are many potential symptoms and signs that may herald the earliest features supporting a diagnosis of Parkinson's disease. It is estimated that a person must lose approximately 60 percent (or more) of the dopamine producing cells in the brain (referred to as the substantia nigra or known in Latin as the black substance), before noticeable changes will be detected. This cell loss always occurs before the symptoms. The threshold of cell loss that must be eclipsed before the appearance of symptoms and this situation can be likened to those who experience kidney failure. When a kidney begins to malfunction, approximately 75 percent or more of its cells are lost, and those cells are unrecoverable. Frustratingly, for kidney failure patients, their routine laboratory tests are almost never abnormal. Just as in Parkinson's disease, there is a threshold of cells that must be lost before one manifests symptoms.

This phenomenon has resulted in scientists turning their attention toward searching for pre-symptomatic screening tests, which have been designed to detect Parkinson's disease prior to the loss of a large number of brain cells. Pre-symptomatic research has focused on areas such as smell testing, constipation, cognitive screening, sleep disorders (acting out one's dreams), imaging, and also blood markers. Currently there is no reliable biomarker for Parkinson's disease, with the exception of the small number of families who carry known genetic mutations. If scientists can manage to develop treatments to retard the progression of symptoms, then early identification through biomarkers will be a critical part of early treatment.

Sometimes the signs of Parkinson's disease are obvious, such as a prominent resting tremor. However, in many instances the symptoms are subtle, and a general doctor may not immediately associate them with Parkinson's disease. (For example, smaller than normal handwriting, called micrographia, shoulder pain, or a decreased arm swing.) The easiest ones to detect are considered to be the common "motor" symptoms (tremor, stiffness, slowness), and these usually occur more prominently on one side of the body. The reason(s) why Parkinson's disease is worse on one side of the body as opposed to the other body side (asymmetric symptoms) remains one of the disease's greatest mysteries[19]. I often joke to the students that if they can figure out why Parkinson's disease presents as an asymmetric entity, they can book their flight to Stockholm, Sweden, and start writing their Nobel address.

The Medication Awakening

Prior to medication therapy, Parkinson's disease patients were placed in asylums because they became stiff and frozen. If all Parkinson's disease patients were institutionalized today, it would break Medicare because there are between one and 1.5 million sufferers in the United States alone.

Institutionalized patients were asked to fold towels and push chart racks for the doctors while they made their daily rounds. Ironically, history would prove that exercise was helpful as a treatment approach. This perspective would emerge decades later as an important "secret" to a happier and life with the disease.

The advent of replacing dopamine (levodopa or sinemet therapy) was a game changer. As illustrated in the 1990 movie "Awakenings," patients woke up and transformed from lifeless statues into full-functioning human beings. Over the years, great expertise has been quickly accumulating on how to address Parkinson's disease pharmacologically, behaviorally, and believe it or not, surgically. There are more than a dozen drugs, multiple behavioral interventions, and several difficult to comprehend but revolutionary surgeries. In many ways, viable treatment options for Parkinson's disease have been significantly ahead of many other neurological diseases.

The "Aha" Moment and Parkinson's Disease

For the patient and the family who expect to go to the doctor and to receive a "million-dollar workup," including blood tests and expensive imaging, then to ultimately have the results packaged into an "aha" diagnostic moment, disappointment will inevitably set in. There is no reliable blood test to diagnose Parkinson's disease, and simple brain MRI testing will currently reveal a bland and normal result. The best way to arrive at a diagnosis of Parkinson's disease is to undergo a neurological examination by an experienced and well-trained neurologist[19]. Your "aha" moment, after a diagnosis of Parkinson's disease should be a well-placed confidence that your journey is not over and that productive years lie ahead.

The first secret to a happier life with Parkinson's disease is simple. The recognition and appreciation of what Parkinson's disease is and is not will form the critical foundation for your journey. Doctors must be, as Tony Dungy says, mentor-leaders and teach their patients the deeper appreciation necessary for progressing to a normal or near normal life for many years to come.

❧ Secret No. 1: Know the Signs

CHAPTER 2:

Timing is Important in Life but Critical in Parkinson's Disease

"The right thing at the wrong time is the wrong thing."
— Joshua Harris

WHETHER YOU ARE GOING TO SEE A MOVIE, running to catch a flight, or have been instructed to take an antibiotic for a potentially life-threatening infection, timing is important. Timing is, however, not just important in Parkinson's disease. It is critical.

Ann Graybiel at the Massachusetts Institute of Technology (MIT) recently discovered that brain cells have a built in timing mechanism[20]. Anne has been on our research board for the National Parkinson Foundation for many years, and she has been a huge advocate of the notion that if we can better understand how and why brain cells keep time, we can develop better approaches to rehabilitation and to treatment.

Our center in Florida has taken care of CEOs of major companies, celebrities, and politicians. However, most of our patients come from main street America. Parkinson's disease patients on average are characterized by being well read. They will follow changes in the therapeutic drug and device pipeline as if they were box scores in a baseball or football game. Because billions of dollars exchange hands between venture capitalists and large industry based companies, The Wall Street Journal will frequently break the news of important therapeutic developments, sometimes even before major medical journals. A major emphasis has been to find the cure. This emphasis may be misplaced. One of the secrets to kindling hope and achieving happiness is not to expect to be cured by pulling a magic lever. The true magic lies in how and when we pull the lever and what we expect to derive from it.

I have been impressed that there is no disease quite like Parkinson's. Oliver Sacks wrote about and Robin Williams starred in a movie about patients who developed Parkinson's disease as a result of one of the famous influenza epidemics[21]. These patients were living locked in asylums until they were administered a pill containing a chemical called dopamine. The patients awoke and came back to life. They walked, they talked, they laughed, and they cried. They visited with family members, and they caught up on a generation lost.

Every time I visit with a new Parkinson's patient, I ask them to come off their dopaminergic drugs. I then carefully examine them and re-administer dopamine in an effort to reproduce an awakening. Joe Friedman, a prominent neurologist from Providence, R.I., taught me many years ago to watch for yawning. The simple yawn is followed by the awakening. Though I have seen this thousands of times, I am still left with a sense of awe, and I am reminded why I love to take care of these patients. The challenge that I issue to every medical student is to name one disease where a pill can completely transform a person from neurologically disabled to normal, often within minutes. To date, no student has won the challenge.

The Frozen Addict

In 1982, George Carillo walked into a California emergency room with the sudden onset of what appeared to be Parkinson's disease. The ER staff was confused. Parkinson's disease was chronic and slowly progressive. How was this possible if just a few hours prior, George was completely normal? Following a dose of levodopa or dopamine replacement therapy he awakened. However, George's story was just beginning to unfold. More suddenly-frozen patients began presenting to emergency rooms with the identical constellation of symptoms, and all improved with the dopamine pill.

Bill Langston, now director of the Parkinson's Institute in Sunnyvale, Calif., would arrive at a startling discovery. Following a good bit of investigative work, Bill uncovered the critical piece of the puzzle. All of the patients had received batches of a designer drug called MPP+. Unfortunately, the chemist who concocted the batches made a slight but important mistake, and the result was that he ended up manufacturing MPTP. MPTP is a chemical that is toxic to the little black dopaminergic cells in the brainstem. These cells are called the substantia nigra, which is Latin for black substance. MPTP is now known worldwide to cause Parkinson's, and the deficits induced by MPTP can be rescued by administering levodopa[22].

You might be thinking to yourself that this MPTP mistake was unfortunate and unacceptable. However, what would you say if I told you that this single tragic mistake has helped more Parkinson's disease researchers than any other discovery since the advent of dopamine replacement therapy itself? The frozen addict led Bill Langston to develop MPTP as a toxin based model. This model closely replicated an animal form of Parkinson's disease. The model is one of the best and most consistent available. Researchers around the world have used Langston's model to unlock many of the secrets of Parkinson's disease. The original California emergency room cases have become famously known as the "frozen addicts."

The Importance of Timing

What Oliver Sacks did not know when he gave his patients dopamine and induced the awakenings was that this long-term strategy would not be enough. One of the most important secrets about Parkinson's disease is that the timing of medication doses is in many cases more important than the dose itself[19]. The timing of when doses are given also changes as the disease progresses, and this is why the most successful Parkinson's disease patients will have a very close relationship with their doctors. An experienced doctor or health care professional can adjust medication regimens and greatly improve the quality of life.

As Parkinson's disease progresses, 80 percent of people will develop a resting tremor, and all sufferers will experience rigidity, slowness, and walking problems. After five years, the majority of patients will have developed medication related on-off fluctuations. In other words, the dopaminergic medication may wear off before the next dose, or alternatively, there may be a delay in reaching a therapeutic blood level of dopamine. Many patients will develop dance-like movement referred to as dyskinesia, and some will suddenly and unexplainably freeze when walking, particularly when traversing doorways or small spaces. Most doctors focus on the dose of medications, and many doctors will follow the knee jerk response to increase the dose regardless of symptoms. Their rationalization for dose escalation may be understandable considering that in most diseases, when medications fade in efficacy, the dose is bumped up. Common examples play out in clinical medicine every day: a seizure patient with a flurry of attacks or a hypertensive patient with elevated blood pressure. In Parkinson's disease, a knee jerk response of increasing medications can sometimes land the patient in an emergency room or even lead to admission to the hospital for uncontrollable movements or hallucinations. In all fairness to general doctors around the world, we should clarify that sometimes the best change is an increase in medication dose. The important point we would like to emphasize is that timing in Parkinson's disease is critical, especially as the disease progresses.

What Oliver Sacks later discovered, as he followed his original cohort of patients, was that increasing the dose was a short-term solution, and long term it resulted in many side effects[21]. He would learn the hard way that Parkinson's disease and Parkinsonian syndromes were complex and that the timing of the medications and also the medication intervals had to be adjusted and tailored for each patient. He also learned that the management of the Parkinson's disease patient was a life-long endeavor. These lessons in the early use of dopamine replacement therapy are frequently lost in busy modern medical practices, but they are still as true as they were more than forty years ago.

It is critical as a patient to remember what I consider to be a cardinal rule of Parkinson's disease management. If your disease is changing and your medication dosages and dosage intervals are not changing to accommodate your symptoms, you may not be medically optimized.

Arguments for Proper Medication Timing

There are other examples where timing is important in Parkinson's disease. One such example is the common mystery of why one leg "freezes" and completely defies the command to move. The brain says go, but the leg won't respond. If the freezing episode coincides during the attempt to turn and move in a different direction, a fall will commonly result[19].

The "tricks" that many patients utilize to break freezing are creative, fascinating, and also relevant to the notion that Parkinson's is a "disease of timing." Counting out loud, marching in place, stepping over an inverted Y-shaped cane or even using a laser pointer have all been utilized to unlock these mysterious freezing episodes.

We treated a race car driver with Parkinson's disease. Interestingly, he did not experience problems operating his car; however he froze in crowds and in the airport. He developed a simple visual cue he used to break his freezing episodes. He bought a laser pointer from Office Depot, and he projected it onto the floor in front of him. When he cued himself to step on the red dot, the freezing disappeared. Later, a company developed a Parkinson's walker with a built in laser pointer. I, like most practicing doctors, lack a keen business sense.

Colum McKinnon at Northwestern University has been researching why patients with Parkinson's disease freeze. He has developed several techniques to treat this phenomenon and also other disabling issues facing Parkinson's disease patients. He and his colleagues recently discovered that startling patients with loud noises could break freezing and also improve movements. McKinnon also observed in a series of important experiments that timing, as Anne Graybiel had argued, was the critical element to improve movement. He and his team have been working on ways to send signals to the brain and to rehabilitate and to improve the lives of Parkinson's disease patients[23, 24].

The second secret to helping Parkinson's disease patients find hope and a happier life is timing. Timing will be an important element to the success or failure of any intervention for the treatment of this disease.

❧ Secret No. 2: Timing is Important in Life, but Timing is Critical in Parkinson's Disease

CHAPTER 3:

Ask Your Doctor if Making Your Brain Electric Would Help Your Parkinson's Disease

"Is it a fact – or have I dreamt it – that, by means of electricity, the world of matter has become a great nerve, vibrating thousands of miles in a breathless point of time?"

— Nathaniel Hawthorne

ALIM BENABID, AN ACCOMPLISHED DOCTOR, was not known beyond his specialized field. He was a professor of neurosurgery at the Joseph Fourier University in Grenoble, France from 1978 to 2007. His routine duties included treating people debilitated by the symptoms of Parkinson's disease by placing small lesions into deep regions within their brains. One day Benabid had a "what if" moment that would forever alter the treatment of Parkinson's disease. More importantly, it would radically and positively impact the lives of many sufferers.

On the operating room table was an elderly man who was afflicted by pain and tremors. Benabid utilized a technique referred to as intraoperative mapping, and as a routine he gathered a detailed physiological brain map. Benabid would obsessively check and double check his map to confirm localization of the "sweet spot." He was aware from his thousands of hours of intraoperative experience that the sweet spot was the precise location within the brain that if tickled would result in relief of Parkinson's symptoms. He also knew that if he missed the spot there would be no relief, and in some cases it could precipitate severe side effects.

Benabid passed a large test probe several centimeters below the brain's surface. Initially, the results were as he predicted; the tremor worsened when he stimulated through the probe with a series of very slow pulses. In contrast, it improved when he stimulated with faster pulses. What happened next was the real breakthrough. Instead of burning a hole in the brain, Benabid decided to change course. It would be hard to not to overstate the significance of this moment because of the tens of thousands of Parkinson's disease and tremor patients whose lives would be forever transformed by that decision. Instead of heating the tip of the test probe and placing a tiny lesion deep inside the brain, he withdrew it and placed what would later be referred to as a DBS lead[25, 26, 27].

Previous to Benabid's use of a chronically implanted DBS lead to treat the symptoms of Parkinson's disease, conventional treatment was to make a brain lesion to "disrupt the disruption" in a rogue brain circuit that was stuck in a state of abnormal oscillation.

One of the amazing observations about the human brain is that its normal functions seem to be dictated by rhythmic oscillations that continuously repeat over and over, much like a popular song on the radio. The oscillations change and modulate and they act to control various human behaviors. If an oscillation "goes bad" it can result in a disabling tremor or alternatively in many of the other symptoms of Parkinson's disease.

That day in the operating room, Alim Benabid decided to remove the lesion probe he had used hundreds of times before and replace it with a wire that had four metal contacts at the tip. This wire, later referred to as a deep brain stimulation (DBS) lead, was connected to an external battery source. Benabid and his neurology colleagues could program the device using a small old-fashioned box with several small buttons and archaic looking switches. As simple as the system appeared, it turned out to be very powerful, allowing Benabid to individualize the settings to a possible 12,000+ combinations. Unlike lesion therapy, this new approach provided Benabid and his team a tailored or personalized medical solution to many of the disabling symptoms of Parkinson's disease and of tremor[25, 26, 27].

There was another potential long-term benefit to Benabid's approach. Patients holding out for stem cells, gene therapy or even a cure, would remain eligible for future operations, since DBS as a therapy was completely reversible. The whole system could be extracted in a small operation that could be performed in a few short minutes. Because of the robust and undeniable benefits of this operation, it would be rare over the next two decades to hear of a patient who would request removal of their DBS device.

Deep Brain Stimulation: The Technology Expands Beyond the Original Vision

As technology has advanced, the term deep brain stimulation has turned out to be less than precise, as the idea of electrical stimulation has led to the development of an entire field sometimes referred to as "neuro-modulation." The reason the term DBS is imprecise is because DBS is not always deep, not always applied in the brain, and doesn't always result in stimulation.

DBS is not limited to the brain as it is now possible to excite and inhibit nerves, nerve coverings, and even the spinal cord. Most people automatically think that the mechanism of action for DBS is stimulation, especially given its name. However, it turns out to be a much more complex and interesting story. Many debates and much research has been generated concerning the potential mechanisms underpinning this technology. Since the effects on humans are so dramatic, it will be critical to understand and unlock how this therapy actually works. Unlocking the secrets of DBS will likely guide the design of more rational drug therapy, gene therapy, and other novel interventions.

The first major debate about DBS occurred between two research groups who lived an ocean apart. The French group that discovered DBS argued that the mechanism of action was blocking or jamming of the brain's electrical activity. The argument they proposed was that DBS acted in an inhibitory way toward cells and toward cell-to-cell connections. Other prominent groups around the world, including Warren Grill at Case Western Reserve University and Cameron McIntyre at the Cleveland Clinic, responded to these early theories by constructing laboratory based models to explain how the electrical current actually interacted with the neurons (brain cells) and with their billions of interconnections, which are referred to as synapses[28, 29, 30, 31, 32, 33]. To virtually everyone's astonishment, it was uncovered that DBS inhibited neurons and excited axons, the pipes extending out from each brain cell. This mind-blowing revelation meant that the mechanism of action for DBS was neither stimulation nor excitation. It was not simply jamming of a brain circuit. DBS was actually affecting a very large network of neural structures up and downstream from a tiny local area of electrical stimulation. This area of delivered electricity, though measuring only a meager three millimeters in diameter, proved to have dramatic effects over the entire brain and body[34].

The early theories of how DBS worked focused on brain cells (neurons) and ignored the supporting cells known as glia and astrocytes. Those supporting cells provide critical infrastructure to facilitate all of the brain's many important functions. As an example of how critical these supporting cells can be, each astrocyte touches as many as two million synapses, which is the term used to describe the brain's interconnections. Synapses facilitate communication and direct information transfer. Forgetting about the supporting cells would be like trying to win a baseball game with only three players on your team. Electricity can act directly on neurons, astrocytes, and synapses, which in turn can propagate a dumping of calcium and subsequently other important brain chemicals such as adenosine and glutamate. The chemicals that get "dumped" in response to electrical modulation are called neurotransmitters. The dumping of these neurotransmitters has emerged as an important element in facilitating the mechanism of action for DBS. It is amazing to think that DBS acts chemically as well as electrically [34, 35, 36].

Since DBS likely works in many ways (electrical, chemical, excitation, and/or jamming inhibition), we now believe that the electrical current sets off a complex symphony of coordinated information transfers between many brain elements and regions. This complex information transfer ultimately leads to improvement in Parkinson's disease symptoms. Since so many regions are involved in this coordinated response, we refer to this as a neural network [34, 37]. Phil Starr, a neurosurgeon at the University of California, San Francisco, has shown that there is a complex relationship between the cells stimulated deep in the brain and the cerebral cortex. When the DBS device is turned on, the cells in the two regions become coherent and fire in a new synchrony.

DBS also stimulates neurogenesis, or the formation of new brain cells. Stimulating the growth of new brain cells has opened up the hope that this technology may unlock better treatments for neurodegenerative diseases such as Parkinson's disease, Alzheimer's disease and Progressive Supranuclear Palsy. Dennis Steindler and colleagues at the University of Florida recently showed that there are neural stem cells in the brains of Parkinson's disease patients, and they can even grow these cells off of discarded DBS leads removed because of device fractures[38, 39]. The cells seem to be drawn to and stick on the DBS lead.

For some of you, DBS may seem like something out of a sci-fi movie, but with all the medical and technological advances that have been recently accomplished, what may seem futuristic has become our new reality. This means that doctors and patients have more treatment options available, and for some who suffer with tremor and the other symptoms of Parkinson's disease, these alternatives can be life changing. New discoveries like DBS that lead to an improvement in disease features have the potential to unlock more of the mystery of Parkinson's disease and lead many patients to happier and more meaningful lives.

The Early Lessons of Neuromodulation for Parkinson's Disease Choosing On Whom to Operate

When we arrived at the University of Florida to build a Parkinson's disease and movement disorders center, there was no basic infrastructure in place for Parkinson's disease care. Dr. Kelly Foote (our neurosurgeon) and I were two "young guns" fresh out of fellowship training. The existing senior faculty made it clear that though they liked us, they were concerned about the potential for trouble, especially with the introduction of a potentially risky neurosurgical procedure. The message to us was: "We like you guys, but don't embarrass us." It was an understandable sentiment, as all seasoned medical school professors over the course of a career will inevitably observe dozens of purported miracle treatments. These types of treatments are usually introduced with glitz and flare, but in the majority of cases they will completely flop. The most concerning issue to our faculty was that we were drilling holes in the skull and poking precious brain tissue. This was much riskier than a simple pill therapy. Their concerns were both understandable and also forgivable.

Over the last ten years at the University of Florida, DBS therapy has transitioned from a crazy notion to a cool procedure and finally to a completely acceptable form of therapy. Every medical student is now required to observe one DBS operation during the course of training. Thanks to Benabid's intraoperative decision and "what if" moment, the world is moving into a bionic age.

A formidable and somewhat unexpected obstacle emerged when we set up the DBS program at our institution. We were faced with an immediate influx of 200 referrals for the procedure. Unfortunately, only eight of these referrals (four percent) were reasonable surgical candidates.

Even more concerning, we observed a few dozen neurosurgeons and hospitals launch ill-fated programs. The field would learn a humbling lesson about the critical importance of choosing the right candidates for DBS. Patient selection would turn out to be the most important factor predicting the success or failure of this relatively new surgical approach. Patients who were inappropriately selected for the surgery often had disappointing and tragic results. Thus, the development of a solid DBS surgical program would require educating primary care and neurology doctors in proper screening and selection techniques, and this effort has been ongoing over the last decade. Also, most neurosurgeons and hospitals would have to inevitably reach the realization that once a Parkinson's patient is implanted, they would likely be bionic for life and would require continuing expert care. Most hospitals were not prepared to organize and invest in this type of interdisciplinary effort. Over the last decade, DBS programs appeared and offered hope to many local and regional patients. However, the majority of these programs quickly faded and ultimately dissolved.

Ironically, DBS drove a worldwide movement toward better interdisciplinary care for the Parkinson's disease patient. Prior to DBS, most care was delivered in isolation by physicians, nurses, nurse practitioners, or physician's assistants. The complexities of screening a DBS candidate would, in contrast to typical care, require a multidisciplinary approach. A neurologist, neurosurgeon, psychologist, radiologist, and psychiatrist would all participate in a comprehensive evaluation. Over time, physical therapists, occupational therapists, speech therapists, and social workers would, as a result of this process, transform into important members of this team. Together the team would make critical surgical decisions, and individually each team member would become an expert in his or her field.

Ultimately, so many people participated in the care of a single DBS patient that the process gradually shifted from multidisciplinary to interdisciplinary. Interdisciplinary care is the highest level of a patient-centric experience, and it has been utilized for decades by cancer centers and rehabilitation hospitals. Interdisciplinary care involves specialists sitting together and discussing an individual patient, which stands in contrast to consultative or multidisciplinary care, where practitioners communicate by sending notes or letters to each other. For Parkinson's disease, the birth of the interdisciplinary DBS evaluation greatly enhanced the level of care and has forged dramatic improvements in patient and family satisfaction. DBS, a surgical not medical procedure, would transform and improve the care for all Parkinson's disease patients, even those not receiving an operation[40, 41, 42].

Brain Mapping

Deep within the research hallways at The Johns Hopkins University, Mahlon DeLong studied a group of circuits referred to as the basal ganglia. His other colleagues and contemporaries in the lab would snatch up the more desirable and easier to decode brain regions. The soft-spoken DeLong would for many years meticulously record and sort single brain cells from Parkinson's disease basal ganglia, first in monkeys, and then in humans. Slowly a coherent picture would begin to emerge, and this picture included important changes in the rate and pattern of brain cell activity[43, 44, 45, 46, 47]. DeLong passed his craft to Jerrold Vitek, Phillip Starr, Thomas Wichmann, Kelly Foote, and many others including myself. We would all spend our careers refining and applying these lessons to the human DBS experience.

The procedure is a marvel of modern medicine. It requires only a dime-sized hole in the skull. The operation is performed in virtual reality on a computer screen and within minutes can be translated into a human patient. The surgeon can navigate around blood vessels and refine a region of interest to reach within a few millimeters of an intended target. A few millimeters may be small on a ruler, but it is very large in brain space. A few millimeters of brain space can be compared to the distance between Florida and California.

A famous neurosurgeon from Toronto named Andres Lozano once declared that mapping a Parkinson's disease patient brain was similar to driving a car through Europe. As the recording microelectrode was advanced one millimeter at a time, the sound of the brain cells changed while moving from one brain region to another. He compared this change to the language changes that can be appreciated when crossing the border from one European country to another. He noted that these changes were instrumental in the process of brain mapping.

After threading several microelectrodes into a Parkinson's disease patient's brain, one can develop a three dimensional map. This map includes both the desired target location and also the position of surrounding brain structures. There are many brain targets that can be chosen for a patient. The choice of target is usually tailored during a detailed discussion, which involves the patient and his or her DBS team. The complete map is a critical part of the DBS procedure itself because if the final DBS lead is misplaced by even a few millimeters, it can be the difference between dramatic success and miserable failure. Failure could mean a lack of benefit, but could also mean that a patient is left with permanent stroke-like symptoms.

Once the final location for the DBS lead has been determined, it can be locked into place by a capping device. A connector wire can be attached and tunneled underneath the skin. In one final step, a battery, referred to as a neurostimulator, can be placed under the collarbone in an identical location. The neurostimulator is like a cardiac pacemaker. Once placed, a neurologist or nurse programmer can cycle through thousands of possible DBS programming parameters in order to optimize the settings for a patient. Optimization of the settings usually takes a few weeks to a few months and can lead to exquisite control of the many disabling symptoms of Parkinson's disease such as tremor, stiffness, slowness, and in some cases even walking[34].

The Dream of Living Pill Free

Most people with Parkinson's disease are fed up with all the medications. In some cases, sufferers may have to take multiple pills every two to three hours around the clock. The price for missing a dose could be tremor, stiffness, slowness, or even falling. In a cruel twist of fate, as

Parkinson's disease progresses, the pills may result in uncontrollable dance-like and flailing movements. These movements have been referred to as dyskinesias, and they occur as a result of disease progression and also a direct result of long-term use of many of the common Parkinson's disease drugs.

When a Parkinson's disease patient takes a dopamine pill a miraculous transformation ensues. Tremor, stiffness, slowness, and many other symptoms melt away within 20 to 30 minutes. A Parkinson's disease sufferer will commonly refer to the period when a pill kicks in as being "on." Conversely, when a dosage drops below a therapeutic blood level and symptoms return, they will refer to this scenario as being "off."

Many Parkinson's disease sufferers will initially respond to the medication, but inevitably and many years later develop medication related on-off fluctuations and dyskinesia. Modern DBS has emerged as the most powerful therapy to address these types of disease related fluctuations. DBS can restore meaningful life in a large number of Parkinson's disease patients.

As the DBS story unfolded in the 1990s, many centers in Europe reported that a patient could completely stop Parkinson's medication. A transoceanic debate ensued with many North American centers advocating a less aggressive approach to medication reduction. Two decades later, the entire field now appreciates that it is very rare to terminate all Parkinson's medications following a DBS operation. We have learned that medication reduction occurs in some but not all patients, and that it is more common when two DBS leads are employed (one on each side of the brain) into a very specific brain region called the subthalamic nucleus. In some cases, apathy, walking problems and other issues will emerge if Parkinson medications are stopped or reduced too quickly. Thus, the hope of offering Parkinson's disease sufferers pill free existences remains largely elusive. Neuromodulation has, however, emerged as a powerful complement to pharmaceutical options and as a means to better manage one's life.

Advancing Technology

One remarkable fact about DBS therapy is that the hardware has changed very little since Benabid's experiment. The brain lead, the connector wires, and the battery technologies have only been slightly improved. The FDA currently has approved only one DBS device for Parkinson's disease patients, and it is well known that better technologies are languishing as they snake their way through the trenches of a difficult FDA approval process. The techniques for delivering currents and for securing the electrodes remain fundamentally unchanged. Despite the lack of a new DBS technology, penetration of the device into communities all over the world has been explosive, with nearly 100,000 Parkinson's and movement disorders patients having been transformed into bionic existences.

Why haven't more DBS devices become available over the past two plus decades? The answer to this question is complex. Studies validating the current DBS technology for Parkinson's disease have revealed clinical outcomes that were more robust than anyone expected. When I entered the field in the mid-to-late 1990s, the top experts advised me against pursuing DBS research, as they were sure the therapy would disappear and be replaced by better medicines. Not only has the therapy survived, but the clinical and financial success of DBS has snowballed, and the effect has drawn more patients, more researchers, and more venture capitalists into the device arena. While many pharmaceutical companies have flirted with the next big Parkinson's drug, none of these efforts have been robust and most have flopped. A multi-billion dollar industry attracts all kinds, and the infusion of novel scientific ideas and fresh cash has brought at least a half a dozen new companies into the electric brain sphere. Each company offers an improvement or tweak to the currently available DBS system, and this is promising for the hope of advancements in the near future.

So what will it take to move the DBS field forward? A critical first step will be to develop an understanding of the needs of the Parkinson's disease sufferers. Patients and families currently seek treatment to address the symptoms that are not adequately covered by medications and current DBS therapy. (For example, thinking issues and falling). Second, the therapy will need to be safe, and clinical trials will need to be sufficiently robust and demonstrate benefit greater than the placebo effect. (For example, improvement greater than would be predicted by chance). Third, the therapy must be cost effective and incrementally better than all existing therapies. Any hope of moving the technology and ultimately the field forward will need to address these three major hurdles.

There have been important and recent research advances in DBS device development. First, there are many new DBS lead designs. Most of the new designs will enable the electrical current to be administered to more specific regions of the brain, thereby enhancing benefits and reducing side effects. Second, the type of electrical current we now utilize is referred to as a voltage-driven system. In this voltage-driven paradigm, there can be shifts over time in the actual size and shape of the electrical field that is delivered to the brain tissue. Newer stimulators will use a constant current device that will smooth tissue delivery and improve the effectiveness of the therapy. A third issue that has emerged is battery life. Clinicians and patients have a critical need for longer lasting, and in some cases, rechargeable batteries. Better battery lives will mean fewer replacement surgeries and less of a chance for battery failure and return of symptoms. These new approaches and products have already begun to appear and are working their way through the FDA approval process.

Patients have also begun to demand sleeker and smaller devices as a box protruding from the chest area is unattractive and undesirable. It would also be preferable to most patients to eliminate the connector wire that attaches the lead in the head to the box in the chest. Finally, it would be ideal to be able to program the device from a remote location. Imagine the day when a doctor can see you by video and tune your device without the need to change out of your pajamas or leave your house. All of these advances are coming soon.

Another encouraging development is the ability to tailor or personalize a therapy for an individual patient. We previously targeted our surgery to one specific area of the brain for all Parkinson's sufferers. With all the advancements, we are able more and more to hone in on specific bothersome symptoms. For example, one brain target may be best for tremor, while another is preferable for speech, and still a third target would be chosen for walking. Patients would choose the target based on their needs (e.g. a chef may choose a target that maximally suppresses tremor, while a trial lawyer or teacher may choose a target that preserves speech). Also, we are no longer limited to one or even two brain leads. The ability to place multiple DBS leads into a single patient over time as his or her disease evolves and new symptoms emerge is quickly becoming a reality.

The Potential for Combining Electricity with Other Therapies

As the mechanisms underpinning the success of the electric brain come into focus, the possibilities and potentials are exploding. Now that we understand that changes in the rate and pattern of neuronal cell firing are responsible for many of the observed benefits, we can harness this information to develop newer and better therapies. Additionally, the realization that many of the clinical benefits result from changes in brain chemicals such as adenosine and glutamate can also help in facilitating the design of more rational drug therapies.

One provocative area of research and development has been the idea to combine DBS with other novel therapies. Specifically, the idea of utilizing a DBS lead as a catheter that can inject genetic therapies, stem cells, and growth factors. The general idea is to combine powerful symptomatic therapy such as brain stimulation with approaches that may have the potential to slow down disease progression. This approach will hopefully offer the best of both worlds.

An Electric Biomarker

The newest Holy Grail in science and in Parkinson's disease will be the development of a biomarker. The National Institutes of Health defines a biomarker as "a characteristic that is objectively measured and evaluated as an indicator of normal biologic processes, pathogenic processes, or pharmacologic responses to a therapeutic intervention." In layman's terms, a biomarker is an indicator that one has or does not have a disease (i.e. a blood test that may reveal the diagnosis of Parkinson's disease). When it comes to the electric brain, scientists have raised the possibility of an electrical biomarker. The general idea is that disease activity could be monitored by an electrical signal that is being naturally emitted by specific brain regions. So instead of using the biomarker to diagnose the disease, doctors would use the abnormal electrical patterns to direct treatment, in this case, electrical treatment of Parkinson's.

It has now become recently possible to record the brain after DBS and capture the signals in real time. Previously, the brain could only be recorded during the actual operating room procedure. The type of signal that can now be collected is called a local field potential or LFP. LFPs are special measurements of the brain's native electrical current and also its inherent oscillatory properties. In Parkinson's disease, research has revealed an important LFP called the beta band. This band changes when medication or DBS is administered. Understanding electrical biomarkers will allow the development of smarter devices. The hope is that new devices will sense a particular abnormality, such as a beta band, and automatically respond. The result is called an on-demand paradigm. In on-demand circuits, electrical abnormalities can be addressed by applying current to the brain. The idea of on-demand systems is to solve brain problems as they emerge and before the development of a particular clinical issue or symptom. Thus the era of personalized medicine has arrived.

❧ Secret No. 3: Ask Your Doctor if Making Your Brain Electric Would Help Your Parkinson's Disease

CHAPTER 4:

Be Aggressive in Treating Depression and Anxiety

"When you're lost in those woods, it sometimes takes you a while to realize that you are lost. For the longest time, you can convince yourself that you've just wandered off the path, that you'll find your way back to the trailhead any moment now. Then night falls again and again, and you still have no idea where you are, and it's time to admit that you have bewildered yourself so far off the path that you don't even know from which direction the sun rises anymore."

— Elizabeth Gilbert

I REMEMBER IN 1987 WHEN THE FDA approved the drug Prozac for addressing the disabling symptoms associated with adult onset depression. The term "Prozac Revolution" was coined and a new treatment era launched. There would be a powerful movement toward aggressively addressing depression and also psychiatric symptoms in the general public. Unfortunately, there was a strong stigma associated with a diagnosis of depression. Most people were embarrassed to communicate to their doctors that they were feeling down or that they were thinking about suicide. The general public considered depression a character flaw and weakness. Insurance carriers imposed "carve outs" with many refusing to cover visits to a psychiatrist or a mental health specialist.

There has been a slow but positive evolution in the thinking about depression over the past two decades. Though many problems still exist in the identification of this common disorder, the social stigma has steadily declined. More drugs have been introduced that have successfully addressed depression and anxiety.

The Worldwide Size of the Depression Problem

The reality of depression in the United States and around the world is that it is common and unavoidable. The majority of people will experience at least one major depressive episode in their lifetime, and as they age many will battle depression.

The Centers for Disease Control and Prevention (CDC) in 2005 estimated that 32,000 suicides per year were occurring in the United States. There were only 18,000 homicides and 12,000 deaths from AIDS. Suicide was listed as the eleventh leading cause of death and narrowly missed the top ten killer list. All experts agree that a critical need exists to better address depression and anxiety and especially to prevent suicide.

The World Health Organization (WHO) measures the global burden of disease and also reports on premature death and disability. The WHO utilizes a measure referred to as the disability adjusted life year or DALY. One DALY is one lost year of healthy life. Neuropsychiatric disease has the greatest number of lost DALYs and overall ranks highest across all disease categories including heart issues, tumors, and injuries. Parkinson's disease depression as a subcategory is ranked sixth in total loss of DALYs. Because of the multi-billion dollar potential, pharmaceutical and device companies have developed a keen interest in the treatment of depression, anxiety, and other neuropsychiatric issues.

As important advances in the treatment of mental illness have emerged, we have improved the overall care for patients with depression and anxiety disorders. In 1940, nearly half a million patients were locked behind the doors of psychiatric facilities and were sentenced to life in an asylum. If you were hospitalized for more than two years, you were likely to remain institutionalized for life. Today these numbers are shrinking especially with improvements in the identification, diagnosis, and appropriate treatment of patients. One measure of the shift in care is the use of antidepressant drugs. Approximately 25 million people in the U.S. will fill a prescription for Prozac this year alone.

Parkinson's Disease Depression

Parkinson's disease depression is common. Many estimates for the number of Parkinson's disease patients with depression exceed half of all diagnosed patients. Most experts agree that at least one third of patients with Parkinson's disease suffer from depression and probably another third suffer from symptoms of depression and do not receive a diagnosis[19].

Most patients with serious depression have one or both of the following symptoms:

- Lack of interest in usual activities and lack of pleasure during favorite activities (also referred to as anhedonia)

- Feelings of hopelessness or generally feeling down in the dumps

Other common symptoms that may be present include:

- Concentration issues

- Low energy

- Feeling tired or fatigued

- Sleep issues

- Waking up early in the morning

- Appetite disturbances

- Decreased desire for sex

- Feelings of worthlessness or guilt

The exact reasons these symptoms commonly emerge in Parkinson's disease patients remain unknown. James Parkinson in his original essay referred to depression and depressive symptoms as melancholia[48, 49, 50]. Many practitioners have in the modern era ignored depression and depressive symptoms in Parkinson's disease and left it unaddressed. Many experts rejected the possibility that it may be a primary symptom of Parkinson's disease rather than a reaction to it.

Several lines of evidence strongly suggest that depression is a primary symptom of Parkinson's disease and not just an emotional reaction. First, depression occurs in Parkinson's disease patients at twice the rate of the general population. Additionally, depression may appear in early, middle, or late stages of the disease, and it typically does not resolve unless treated. The most convincing evidence that depression in Parkinson's disease is a real entity has been revealed through results from brain imaging studies and postmortem brain samples. These types of studies have aided in proving the hypothesis that Parkinson's disease is more than a disease of dopamine deficiency. These studies have revealed profound deficits in serotonin, norepinephrine, and acetylcholine. Deficiencies in all three of these chemicals have been strongly associated with the degenerative process[51, 52, 53].

An important secret in the successful management of Parkinson's disease is early identification and aggressive treatment of depression and also of depressive symptoms. Each patient requires an individualized short and long-term treatment plan. In all cases, dopaminergics should be optimized as under medication or not taking doses frequently enough may result in depression or depressive symptoms. In some cases, patients will even describe depression, anxiety, or both when weaning off of their medications between their prescribed dosage intervals. In mild cases of depression, the addition of a medicine may be sufficient (e.g.

serotonin reuptake inhibitors, tricyclic antidepressants, or serotonin and norepinephrine reuptake inhibitors)[19]. It is important to be clinically examined by your doctor four to six weeks after initiation of therapy to ensure the dose was appropriate and that there were no treatment limiting side effects. Herb Ward, a psychiatrist at UF, pointed out to me that neurologists do a poor job in immediately following up with their patients after initiating an antidepressant. This is an area where we all need to improve.

In addition to medication therapy, I usually address sleep issues and whenever possible utilize counseling. In cases where depression is moderate to severe, I will immediately involve a psychiatrist. Communication is critical as some psychiatric medications may worsen Parkinson's disease (e.g. dopamine blockers). Additionally, we always assess suicidal tendencies and advise immediate medical attention if present. I try to remind severely depressed Parkinson's disease patients that though it may seem hopeless, with appropriate treatment they will likely improve and resume a happier and more meaningful life.

Severe depression resistance to medications and also resistance to counseling therapy may be addressed by electroconvulsive therapy (ECT), vagus nerve stimulation (VNS), transcranial magnetic stimulation (TMS), and deep brain stimulation (DBS). TMS and DBS are more experimental but can be options in more experienced centers. ECT, though stigmatized by movies such as "One Flew Over the Cuckoo's Nest" starring Jack Nicholson, has been shown to be very effective therapy for patients who are resistant to medications and counseling.

DBS and New Therapies for Depression

At our center, Herb Ward and Kelly Foote, our neurosurgeon, have been tickling a region of the brain with a DBS lead. It is an improbable combination seeing a psychiatrist and neurosurgeon working together, but it is evidence of how far the field has come in the last 50 years. The region of the brain they have been interested in is area 25. Many years ago a neuroscientist named Korbinian Brodmann assigned each region of the brain a number. Area 25 was shown by a neurologist named Helen Mayberg at Emory University to be an important center modulating human sadness. She elegantly lit up this area of the brain using functional MRI scanning. Her studies revealed that both antidepressants and DBS have the potential to reverse brain abnormalities in this area and, in carefully selected patients, that these therapies can improve quality of life. Though DBS therapy is not ready for prime time in Parkinson's disease, patients should remember that scientists and clinicians are making strides in treating what previously seemed to be impossibly refractory mood disorders.

Anxiety and Panic in Parkinson's Disease

It has been estimated that thirty to forty percent of patients with Parkinson's disease may suffer from anxiety. Common symptoms of anxiety include excessive and constant worrying, feeling nervous, and general inner feelings of terror. Many patients have described these inner feelings as if their life is out of control or that they feel overwhelmed. Other common anxiety symptoms may include[54]:

- Problems sleeping

- Problems concentrating

- A feeling as if the heart is racing

- A feeling of inner restlessness

- Sweating

- Nausea or stomach upset

- Shortness of breath

A subset of patients with Parkinson's disease will also experience panic attacks. A panic attack is marked by short periods of an intense feeling of generalized discomfort or of overwhelming fear. These episodes usually begin abruptly and may last as long as an hour. During a panic attack, the sufferer may feel a sense of doom or as though something bad is about to happen or even experience an uncontrollable fear of dying. Other common symptoms of panic attacks include a feeling that the heart is racing, dizziness, nausea, and sometimes even sweating. An important piece of information is that one-third of Parkinson's disease patients may have anxiety, but one-fifth of Parkinson's caregivers will also have anxiety. Since depression commonly occurs in caregivers, you should be sure to arrange for treatment of caregivers as well as patients. A happy caregiver usually translates to a happy Parkinson's disease patient.

Treatment of anxiety is trickier than depression, and in some instances the two will coincide. Most experienced practitioners will determine whether the anxiety is associated with the "off" dopaminergic medication state. If anxiety worsens or occurs only when the patient is in an "off" medication phase, treatment may focus on moving medication intervals closer together. In some cases, doses will be increased. Anxiety occurring in an optimally-treated Parkinson's disease patient is a more difficult entity to address. It is usually practical to involve a psychiatrist and to determine if the patient possesses a generalized anxiety disorder or another anxiety syndrome. The first line for pharmacotherapy is serotonin reuptake inhibitors, serotonin norepinephrine reuptake inhibitors, and tricyclic antidepressants. For generalized anxiety disorder and more severe cases of anxiety, we will typically add buspirone and possibly a benzodiazepine. Be careful with benzodiazepines (diazepam, clonazepam, Xanax), as their use has been linked to an increased risk of falling. Other good treatments include counseling, cognitive behavioral therapy, as well as Qi Gong and Tai Chi[19].

The Sobering Reality of Untreated Mood Disorders in Parkinson's Disease

Laura Marsh, a psychiatrist at Baylor University performed a very important NIH study when she was at Johns Hopkins University. Laura went into community practices to study Parkinson's disease depression, anxiety, and other neuropsychiatric manifestations. What she found could be considered shocking. The majority of Parkinson's disease patients are suffering from potentially treatable mood disorders, and we need to identify and treat them[55, 56, 57, 58]. Additionally, many more Parkinson's disease patients suffer from plain apathy than from depression as was recently shown by Dawn Bowers and her colleagues at the University of Florida[59]. Apathy, if present, should also be addressed. This secret will undoubtedly lead more people to happier and more meaningful lives.

❧ Secret No. 4: Be Aggressive in Treating Depression and Anxiety

CHAPTER 5:

Sleep Away Your Problems

We need to convince 100 percent of the public, rather than just 40 percent, that good sleep is as necessary as exercise and nutrition for optimal health."
— Robert Schriner, M.D.

ONE OF THE GREAT LESSONS that we have learned over the past decade has been that sleep disorders in Parkinson's disease are common, treatable, and under appreciated. There has, in general, been an over emphasis on easily recognizable Parkinson's symptoms such as tremor, stiffness, slowness, and walking problems, and this has distracted many doctors from even asking their patients about sleeping issues. Lack of sleep in Parkinson's disease will lead to a next day that is dominated by fatigue, irritability, and often feelings of depression.

How common are sleep disorders in Parkinson's disease? Studies have consistently demonstrated that sleep disorders occur in more than two thirds of Parkinson's disease sufferers. They include excessive daytime sleepiness, insomnia, night-time motor symptoms, and also sleep-related breathing disorders (i.e. apnea)[19, 60, 61, 62, 63].

Patients and families should be aware of the possible underlying causes of sleep disorders. The degeneration or loss of cells in the brain may result in sleep dysfunction. Alternatively, the Parkinson's disease symptoms may emerge at night, and tremor, stiffness, and slowness may disrupt sleep. Finally, patients and families must keep in mind that medications, both Parkinson's and non-Parkinson, may impact sleep.

There are a few important rules to follow when addressing sleep disorders in Parkinson's disease patients. The most important rule is to establish the diagnosis. Therapy selection will critically depend on the exact nature of the sleep disorder. It is a myth that a sleeping pill is the treatment for all forms of insomnia. More than one treatable issue can affect sleep, and in complex cases, multiple issues can cloud the overall picture. For example, depression and early morning awakenings may exist in the setting of another sleep disorder. The second rule is not to hesitate to undergo an overnight sleep study. This simple test, which is video recorded, will usually unlock the mystery of the underlying sleeping problem and also any associated movement or breathing issues. Too often a general practitioner or a neurologist will push dosages of sleeping medications higher instead of simply establishing the correct diagnosis prior to proceeding with treatment.

The final issue that must be addressed is to comprehensively review the medication list. This review should include Parkinson's and non-Parkinson-related medications. Dopamine agonists have been associated with sleep dysfunction in Parkinson's disease; however, in some cases levodopa can also lead to fatigue and sleeping issues. We have encountered cases when a dose of levodopa was slowly increased over many years to treat worsening Parkinson's symptoms, and fatigue and sleepiness became an emergent issue. Ramon Rodriguez, a former fellow and now colleague at UF, once embarrassed me by reducing the medications on one of my extremely fatigued, long-standing patients. He eliminated the man's disabling fatigue, and in the process humbled me, teaching me an important lesson I never forgot.

In summary, there are five main sleep issues that you should talk with your doctor about.

1. Insomnia- The inability to fall asleep or sleeping only a few hours at a time.

2. Excessive daytime sleepiness (EDS)- Falling asleep during the day, sleep attacks, fatigue (watch out for medications as a potential cause, particularly dopamine agonists and pain medications).

3. Periodic limb movements- Slow rhythmic movements of the legs and feet while sleeping (picked up on a video-recorded sleep study); Restless legs- An inner feeling of restlessness that requires the sufferer to move his or her legs to resolve the uncomfortable feeling.

4. Rapid eye movement sleep behavior disorder (RBD)- Normally during dream sleep all human muscles are calm. In this disorder there may be vivid dreams and acting out of dreams, which may lead to self injury or injury to a bed partner. The most common treatment is a benzodiazepine such as clonazepam.

5. Sleep related breathing disorders- The most common is sleep apnea where the sufferer may not realize they have pauses in breathing. This may lead to many awakenings during the night and can erode sleep quality.

One of the most common and also heartbreaking stories typically comes from the spouse and not the patient. Spouses will describe their Parkinson's partners as acting out dreams and in many cases "fighting the bad guys." This unfortunately in many cases leads a Parkinson's disease patient to inadvertently strike his or her spouse during dream sleep (REM sleep behavioral disorder). This can understandably lead to marital strife and sleeping in separate beds. This problem is easily addressable by prescribing a bedtime low dose of a drug called a benzodiazepine (e.g. clonazepam, lorazepam, diazepam).

Another heartbreaking story is of a Parkinson's disease patient who has been disabled by fatigue for more than ten years. Following a simple overnight sleep study, it is revealed that they are suffering from apnea. In sleep apnea, the sufferer unconsciously stops breathing, sometimes more than a hundred times an hour. This leads the Parkinson's patient to drift in and out of sleep and ultimately to suffer from fatigue during the day. Treatment with a breathing machine called CPAP (continuous positive airway pressure), usually resolves the issue, and eliminates the daytime fatigue[19, 60, 61, 62, 63].

Depression and Sleep Hygiene

Additionally, you should be assessed and if necessary treated for depression, anxiety, or other affective disorders, as these may contribute to worsening of sleep. Many people remain unaware of the strong connection between mood and sleep, and Laura Marsh found this in her NIH study. Waking up early in the morning may be a sign of untreated depression; however, one should also keep in mind that extra doses of levodopa at night will sometimes also improve sleep quality by suppressing re-emergent Parkinson's disease symptoms.

Sleep hygiene refers to the identification and treatment of behavioral and environmental factors that may affect sleep. Here are some general recommendations that have helped many Parkinson's patients over the years.

- Strive for seven or more hours of sleep each night

- Realize that sleeping more than nine hours can lead to excessive daytime somnolence

- Eliminate alcohol within a few hours of bed time

- Reduce caffeine (coffee, teas, sodas, chocolates) after dinner and prior to bed time

- Create a dark and comfortable sleeping space

- Eliminate television and electronic media devices from the sleeping space

- Exercise every day but not after dinner

❧ Secret No. 5- Sleep Away Your Problems

CHAPTER 6:

Addiction-like Symptoms Can Emerge in Parkinson's Disease

"People should watch out for three things: avoid a major addiction, don't get so deeply into debt that it controls your life, and don't start a family before you're ready to settle down."

—James Taylor

FOLLOWING THE INTRODUCTION OF PILLS containing dopamine for the treatment of Parkinson's disease there was a brief period when medical experts and patients all believed the miracle cure had arrived. Previously, sufferers were frozen like statues and often institutionalized. After taking dopamine pills, they were walking again and were observed to be free of the burdens of Parkinson's disease. It did not take long for scientists to better understand that dopamine pills were only a symptomatic treatment, and that the pills would fall short of preventing the disease from progressing. Additionally, a few years into dopamine treatment, the majority of patients would begin to report complications such as wearing off and also extra movements which have been referred to as dyskinesia.

Addiction-Like Behaviors and Levodopa Therapy

Andre Barbeau published a series of articles in the early to mid 1970s reporting on the benefits and complications of levodopa therapy. Barbeau observed several patients with unusual side effects as a result of dopamine replacement. He reported that more than half of his patients that were placed on very high doses of dopamine (four to six grams a day) appeared manic or hyped up. He also observed that a handful of patients became hypersexual, developed personality issues, and had faulty judgment when making major decisions[64, 65, 66, 67, 68].

Punding

Later, Joe Friedman and colleagues at Brown University discovered that patients on levodopa could also pund[69, 70]. Punding was first described by G. Rylander in 1972 in patients suffering from amphetamine overdose or toxicity. The phenomenon of punding was actually first described in the World War II novel "Catch-22" by Joseph Heller[71].

The story has become famous. "Catch-22" illustrated that a concern for one's safety in the face of dangers that were real and immediate was the process of a rational mind. Orr, a pilot and one of the main characters, was crazy and could be grounded. All he had to do was ask. As soon as he did, he would no longer be crazy and he would have to fly more missions. Orr would be crazy to fly more missions and sane if he didn't, but if he were sane he had to fly them. If he flew them, he was crazy and didn't have to, but if he didn't want to, he was sane and had to. Yossarian was moved very deeply by the absolute simplicity of this clause of "Catch-22" and let out a respectful whistle.[72]"

—Joseph Heller, Catch-22

The Oxford English Dictionary defines a catch-22 as a "set of circumstances in which one requirement, etc., is dependent upon another, which is in turn dependent upon the first."

"Catch-22" was written about a World War II flier named John Yossarian. The pilot tries to survive the war while living under a catch-22. In Chapter 3, "Havermayer," Yossarian returns from the infirmary. He discovers fellow bombardier Orr performing an unusual behavior.

"Orr, who, on the day Yossarian came back, was tinkering with the faucet that fed gasoline into the stove he had started building while Yossarian was in the hospital. "What are you doing?" Yossarian asked guardedly when he entered the tent, although he saw at once. "There's a leak here," Orr said. "I'm trying to fix it."

"Orr was kneeling on the floor of the tent. He worked without pause, taking the faucet apart, spreading all the tiny pieces out carefully, counting and then studying each one interminably as though he had never seen anything remotely similar before, and then reassembling the whole small apparatus, over and over and over and over again, with no loss of patience or interest, no sign of fatigue, no indication of ever concluding.[72]"

This behavior is called punding, and the phenomenon occurs in a select group of patients on levodopa and sometimes on dopamine agonists. "Punding" is an intense fascination with repetitive manipulation of technical or mechanical equipment, the continued handling, examining, and sorting of common objects, grooming, hoarding, abnormally increased writing, and even excessive non-socially sanctioned dancing. [69, 70, 71]"

In Parkinson's disease I have seen punders do all sorts of unusual and repetitive activities including assembling and disassembling watches, fishing, painting, emailing, and ripping out magazine pages. Attempts to stop the stereotyped behaviors are usually met with resistance, irritability, and mood changes. The sufferer would in many cases rather urinate on him or herself rather than stop the behavior. Some caregivers actually prefer the punding state, as the sufferer is usually safe, engaged, and satisfied.

Punding was first described in the medical literature by Rylander et al. in 1972. Joseph Heller wrote "Catch-22" in the early 1950s, and the novel was published in 1961, 11 years before Rylander's description.

Therefore, the novel actually preceded the appreciation of this behavioral phenomenon. In Heller's novel the punding is a result of a head injury that was inflicted by the heel of a stiletto from an Italian prostitute. In Parkinson's disease, punding can result from dopamine replacement or dopamine agonist therapy[71].

All Parkinson's disease patients or caregivers should alert his or her doctor if any unusual behavior arises during dopaminergic treatment. Unusual behaviors including punding may be treatable by simple adjustments in medications or by adding other pharmacological agents such as quetiapine, clozapine, or even a mood stabilizer[19].

Dopamine Dysregulation Syndrome

A rare issue that may occur while using dopamine replacement therapy (e.g. Sinemet or Madopar) is called the dopamine dysregulation syndrome. Andrew Lees and his colleagues at Queen's Square Hospital in London have also referred to this as the hedonistic homeostatic dysregulation syndrome.[73]. The symptoms manifest rarely in only about one to three percent of patients taking dopamine replacement therapy, and the original descriptions focused only on Sinemet (European) and Madopar. It is believed to be an addiction-like syndrome, as patients will crave their medications and consume large quantities of them despite any ill effects. The medications are thought to stimulate the reward centers in the brain, thus the reason that it may be difficult for clinicians to address. Treatment has been comprised of medication adjustments, cognitive behavioral therapy, and also counseling. Also, like in punding, quetiapine, clozapine, or a mood stabilizer may be helpful in restoring a normal life.

Sinemet and Madopar are Not Toxic

Dopamine agonists were introduced in the 1990s as a potential alternative or adjunctive treatment to accompany dopamine replacement therapy (e.g. levodopa). These drugs were sold to the public with suggestions that they would possibly slow disease progression and their use would result in fewer complications when compared to levodopa. Many of the original claims attacking levodopa were driven by an over-exuberant pharmaceutical industry that was looking to displace levodopa as the mainstay of Parkinson's disease therapy. The effects of this anti-levodopa campaign have been felt worldwide, though it is now recognized that there are more side effects and more issues associated with agonist use and that levodopa is an excellent drug for the treatment of Parkinson's disease.

Many Parkinson's disease patients and families members have been unnecessarily alarmed by the continuing reports that Sinemet and/or Madopar may accelerate disease progression. Many neurologists have unneccesarily limited doses and drug intervals. The reports have been fueled by almost non-existent human-based evidence. Patients and families should be aware that dopamine replacement therapies such as Sinemet and Madopar remain the single most effective and important treatment for Parkinson's disease.

Dopamine replacement therapy is not toxic, and does not accelerate disease progression. Laura Parkkinen and colleagues at Queen Square in London examined the pathology in 96 post-mortem Parkinson's disease brains and paired the tissue with clinical information including information on levodopa use. The study concluded that in the human condition "chronic use of L-dopa did not enhance progression of Parkinson's pathology."

In an accompanying editorial, prominent neurologists in the field pointed out that there "remained lingering concerns as to whether levodopa was toxic to dopamine neurons and accelerates the degenerative process." The science used to support these claims included levodopa undergoing auto-oxidation and forming reactive oxygen species and also the presence of toxic protofibrils. Additionally, the proof included an experiment in which levodopa was mixed with brain cells and placed in a dish. The levodopa in the dish was toxic to the brain cells also contained in the dish. The research, however, fell short in demonstrating the toxicity of the drug in the human form of Parkinson's disease.[74, 75]

There are multiple levels of evidence from numerous studies drawn from many countries. Most recently and prominently was the ELLDOPA study, which was published by Stanley Fahn from Columbia University in New York. Stan is one of the founders of modern movement disorders neurology, and he concluded that levodopa was extremely beneficial to the human patient and that it had a possibly positive—not negative—effect on the disease course[76]. There is now a follow-up study being conducted in the Netherlands by Rob de Bie that will likely provide even more evidence of the benefits of levodopa therapy.

Sinemet was recently reported as the most commonly administered drug among more than 6,000 patients being followed longitudinally in the National Parkinson Foundation Quality Improvement Initiative study, also called the Parkinson Outcome Project[77]. It is the largest and longest running Parkinson's disease study ever attempted. Expert practitioners in this study were shown to utilize levodopa more than any other drug, including dopamine agonists, and they used levodopa more as the disease durations increased. Patients should keep all of this information in mind if a practitioner is trying to talk them out of levodopa.

What all this adds up to for patients and for Parkinson's sufferers is that Sinemet and Madopar should be considered safe and effective as treatments for Parkinson's disease. The doses and intervals should be frequently adjusted by an experienced neurologist or practitioner in order to maximize benefits and tailor the therapy to individual symptoms. Patients and families should keep in perspective that the talk about levodopa being toxic and accelerating disease progression can become a major distraction to good care practices. Precious minutes in the doctor-patient relationship should not be wasted on these claims, and prescribers should not under-dose this critical therapy, especially in patients with treatable symptoms. Critics of Sinemet and Madopar will need to bring forward much stronger human data if they wish to change clinical practice. In the mean time, we need to serve our patients by sharing with them the weight of the evidence that strongly supports that levodopa replacement therapy is not toxic and does not accelerate Parkinson's disease progression[19].

Serious Emerging Risks of Addictive-Like Behaviors and Dopamine Agonists

Additionally, we now understand there are serious risks that may be associated with dopamine agonists and that serious complications may occur in almost one in six people taking this class of drugs[78, 79, 80, 81, 82]. Physicians, family members and patients should understand the potential risks of dopamine agonists before they undergo a trial of these medications with patients. Though the effects of agonists can be positive and are actually positive for the majority of sufferers, when compulsive and impulsive issues emerge, agonists can fuel damaging behavior that can wreak havoc on families, as has been pointed out by Tony Lang at Toronto Western Hospital. Tony is one of the world's top leaders in the field, and his voice matters. If patients and families are aware of the risks of agonists, they can quickly discontinue or replace the therapy if problems are encountered.

The development of impulse control disorders as a result of the use of dopamine agonists has become a huge issue in clinical practice and also a very large legal issue with multiple class action lawsuits. Dan Weintraub, M.D., of the University of Pennsylvania, Philadelphia studied 3,090 patients being treated for Parkinson's disease at 46 movement disorder centers in the United States and Canada. Dan and his colleagues identified impulse control issues in a surprising 13.6 percent of patients, including gambling in 5 percent, compulsive sexual behavior in 3.5 percent, compulsive buying in 5.7 percent, binge eating disorder in 4.3 percent and two or more of those issues emerging in 3.9 percent. The most important point for patients to remember is that the disorders were more common in individuals taking dopamine agonists when compared with patients not taking dopamine agonists (17.1 percent vs. 6.9 percent)[81].

A profile emerged for those at risk for these behaviors following the use of agonists. Dan cited being younger or unmarried, smoking cigarettes, and having a family history of gambling problems as important issues to uncover prior to starting an agonist[81, 82].

In 2007, Hubert Fernandez, now the chief of movement disorders at Cleveland Clinic, and I shared a medical student named Mike Shapiro. Mike went into psychiatry, but he published an important paper called "The four As associated with pathological Parkinson disease gamblers: anxiety, anger, age, and agonists." These behaviors included dopamine agonist use, age (young), anxiety, and anger[83]. We unfortunately left out the fifth A, which is a history of alcohol or substance abuse as later pointed out by Valerie Voon, a psychiatrist at Cambridge University in the United Kingdom[78, 79]. It is critical that doctors and patients understand the risk profile for the development of impulse control disorders prior to prescribing dopamine agonists for any patient with Parkinson's disease.

Dopamine agonists have been increasingly used to treat other conditions such as restless legs syndrome, prolactinomas, and fibromyalgia. There is now evidence that these drugs may result in impulse control issues in these other non-Parkinson's disease-related patient groups.

In 2011, one of our fellows in training from Thailand, Natlada Limotai, wrote a very important article about dopamine dysregulation, punding, impulse control disorders, and the dopamine agonist withdrawal syndrome (DAWS)[84]. Our clinical group was becoming increasingly concerned that the word about addictive-like behaviors in Parkinson's disease was not getting out. Each year at NPF we were receiving an increasing number of letters from patients and family members who reported that there were devastating life effects associated with the use of dopamine agonists. I was also seeing the same issues unfold in my personal practice at the University of Florida. Marriages were breaking up, and there were too many cases of hypersexuality, binge eating, compulsive internet use, and compulsive internet pornography to chalk up to chance. At the same time, however, we were bumping up against serious resistance from neurologists and general practitioners who refused to accept the possibility that addiction may occur in Parkinson's disease patients. We worked very hard to publish a paper reviewing our nine-year experience and make it widely available to the public and the medical profession. We purposely titled the paper "Addiction-like manifestations and Parkinson's disease: a large single center 9-year experience," as we wanted to directly confront the myth that addiction could not occur in the setting of Parkinson's disease.

Natlada reviewed more than 1,000 patient charts and found that eight percent of patients who tapered dopamine agonists developed a dopamine agonist withdrawal syndrome (DAWS) that was similar to syndromes reported in opioid and cocaine users[84]. The idea of DAWS was first introduced by Melissa Nirenberg during her movement disorders fellowship training at Cornell University in New York. Melissa picked up on the existence of the withdrawal syndrome by simply listening to her patients that were calling in with complaints that sounded like withdrawal symptoms[85]. It was a keen and important observation.

Natlada reported that about one percent of her sample had the dopamine dysregulation syndrome, which is the syndrome associated with levodopa or dopamine pill addiction. The largest number of behavioral issues in her series, however, occurred with impulse control disorders (ICDs), which were present in nine percent of subjects. The actual rates were underestimated, however, as the most recent series reports about 14 percent. We reasoned that the low numbers were artificial and caused by a lack of awareness in the first nine years of the study. We simply missed their occurrence! Interestingly, punding was seen in both impulse control disorder patients and dopamine dysregulation patients[84]. We were able to conclude, like Dan Weintraub, Valerie Voon, Tony Lang, many other leading authorities, that dopaminergic therapy in Parkinson's disease patients was strongly associated with addiction-like behavioral issues in a surprisingly large subset of patients.

Treatment

Reducing or discontinuing dopamine agonists, as well as adding other medications to block behavioral issues, has been the mainstay of therapy for these addictive-like manifestations. Counseling and cognitive behavioral therapy have been suggested as treatment approaches but have yet to be carefully studied. Some groups have even suggested the use of a surgical technique, deep brain stimulation. The treatment presumption was that by adding deep brain stimulation, patients would be able to reduce dopaminergic medications and therefore combat the addiction-like manifestations.

One of our medical students, Sarah Moum, recently took a look back through the medical records of all of our patients who had DBS surgery. There was no change in dopamine dysregulation diagnosis following either unilateral or bilateral stimulation of any brain target (subthalamic nucleus or globus pallidus internus). Two of seven impulse control patients reported that their symptoms resolved, however, there was a post-operative development of impulse control issues in 17 patients and also post-operative development of dopamine dysregulation in two patients. The lesson learned was that ICDs and DDS should be addressed prior to a DBS operation and that DBS not a primary treatment and can precipitate problems[86]. A group from Grenoble, France, led by Paul Krack has recently introduced a methodology whereby it may be safer to apply DBS to those suffering from ICDs[87].

❧ Secret No. 6: Addiction-like Symptoms Can Emerge in Parkinson's Disease

CHAPTER 7:

Exercise Improves Brain Function

Lack of activity destroys the good condition of every human being, while movement and methodical physical exercise save and preserve it.

—Plato

MANY YEARS BEFORE ADEQUATE MEDICATION treatments were developed to address the various symptoms of Parkinson's disease, some doctors recommended exercise, staying busy, and trying to be as "physical" as possible. There are stories of institutionalized Parkinson's disease patients (prior to the levodopa era) who were asked to push the chart cart for doctors on rounds or fold towels for hospital staff. Early observations about improvements in Parkinson's disease patients following task-specific physical exertion have contributed to the belief that exercise may be beneficial. For years, in my own practice, I have expressed to patients that exercise is "like a drug" and that a daily stretching and exercise routine may be of significant benefit. I have also noticed that patients who receive physical therapy in the hour prior to their appointment with me frequently seem brighter and more optimistic. Though I personally believe in exercise for Parkinson's sufferers, we have, until recently, lacked a strong scientific rationale to prescribe it.

The Evidence for Exercise

Michael Zigmond, Ph.D., at the University of Pittsburgh and a renowned neuroscientist reviewed the topic of whether exercise could be neuroprotective or even disease-modifying in Parkinson's disease patients. Mike was instrumental in uniting clinicians and researchers to move this field forward, and he was involved in many early experiments. His group studied the effects of exercise in a 6-hydroxydopamine animal model of Parkinson's disease. When Mike forced the animals to exercise, he observed that the exercise reduced their vulnerability to developing Parkinson's disease symptoms. Mike speculated that exercise increased chemicals in the brain known as trophic factors and that these trophic factors protected brain cells from dying[88, 89].

Beth Fisher, Giselle Petzinger, and colleagues at the University of Southern California in Los Angeles have moved the research on exercise in Parkinson's disease from animal models into human studies. They published an article in the Archives of Physical Medicine and Rehabilitation that aimed to "obtain preliminary data on the effects of high-intensity exercise on functional performance in people with Parkinson's disease." They also wanted to determine whether improved performance was accompanied by positive physiological alterations in the brain. The results revealed a modest improvement in the motor subscale for Parkinson's disease (called the UPDRS). High intensity exercise had the greatest benefits. The findings supported symptomatic benefits from exercise, particularly with high intensity exercise. This study, along with several other recent studies, has changed clinical practice as most movement disorders experts now tell their patients to exercise every day[90, 91].

Large studies are needed to address whether the symptomatic benefits of exercise will also translate to a decrease in falling. Thankfully there are many studies either nearing completion or publication. These include Daniel Corcos, Christopher Hass, and David Vaillancourt's studies on resistance training in Parkinson's disease. Additionally, several other studies have been published including one in the New England Journal of Medicine touting Tai Chi as a treatment for balance issues[92, 93].

Anke Snijders and Bastiaan Bloem recently reported on a remarkable Parkinson's disease patient in a short report also published in the New England Journal of Medicine. The case was accompanied by a dramatic video that revealed a late-stage Parkinson's disease patient with severe ambulation difficulties and also freezing of gait. The patient had Parkinson's disease for many years, but he reported being able to mount and ride a bicycle for six or more miles each day. This struck Dr. Bloem as "very interesting."[94, 95]

One thing I have personally learned over many years of caring for Parkinson's disease patients is to trust what a Parkinson's disease patient says. Bloem and colleagues did the right thing by pursuing and verifying this story. Their dramatic report actually followed in the wake of another observation made by Jay Alberts, Ph.D., from the Georgia Institute of Technology and later the Cleveland Clinic Foundation. Jay demonstrated that tandem biking and forced exercise was beneficial in Parkinson's disease[96]. His observation was made while tandem biking with a Parkinson's disease patient in the rear seat. He performed this bike ride for charity, and he did it all the way across Iowa. The patient was remarkably improved by the tandem ride. Jay was at Georgia Tech when I was at Emory in Atlanta, and we both shared this same patient but for different research protocols. My protocol was a massive failure. Jay's, however, led to a trek across Iowa and an important breakthrough in Parkinson's disease exercise-based research.

Why does cycling improve symptoms? Why could Bloem's patient ride a bicycle but not walk? These answers remain a mystery, but many experts believe the answer may lie deep in the brain within a group of highly complex and interconnected structures (i.e. the basal ganglia). This network of structures aids in the facilitation of motor, mood, and cognitive functions. How the basal ganglia works remains one of humankind's greatest mysteries. We believe these systems act as advanced data processors and function in modulating complex brain functions and also by filtering and sorting information. Perhaps it was the basal ganglia itself that facilitated the man described by Bloem as able to ride a bike but unable to walk.

Alternatively, the basal ganglia may have been bypassed by other brain systems in order to facilitate his amazing ride. Basal ganglia diseases (e.g. Parkinson's or other movement disorders) are known to be worsened by stress and anxiety (e.g. sleep deprivation or marital issues) but are also known to be improved by mood, exercise, visual/other cues, as well as many non-pharmacological and non-surgical modalities (e.g. Tai Chi). We need to learn more about how the basal ganglia works, and we need to understand how to harness the power of exercise therapy[97].

Bloem, in a recent interview with the New York Times, noted that he "was not advocating that Parkinson's disease patients hop on bikes and go out on busy roads." He clarified that the patients will need help in mounting a bike and that they can get into trouble if they have to stop at traffic lights. They need to ride in safe areas. He recommended that patients ride tricycles or use stationary bikes or trainers—devices that turn road bikes into stationary ones. He also intimated that in select patients "bicycling offers an opportunity to be symptom-free and to get some real cardiovascular exercise, even when their disease is so far advanced that they cannot walk."

The Bloem observation remains interesting, but I want to caution all patients with Parkinson's disease not to jump the gun and try it. Remember, Bloem is from the Netherlands where virtually everyone rides bikes over their entire lifetime. Sudden medication offs, balance problems, and other complex issues could lead to crashes and severe injury. It is best to seek the advice of a doctor and physical therapist, and if you choose to ride into the sunset on your new bicycle, do it with a buddy and a helmet.

The NPF Center of Excellence in the Netherlands is led by Bloem and Martin Munneke. They introduced the ParkinsonNet concept to the field. ParkinsonNet is a framework that was created and intended for igniting a sea change in Parkinson's-related care. The concept is powerful and potentially able to be modified and exported to other regions and countries. The idea is simple: deliver Parkinson's disease care through an integrated network (that may be geographically dispersed across a country) that would provide a more convenient and more integrated experience for patients. Bloem and Munneke performed a trial of almost 700 patients within community-based hospitals. They assigned patients to ParkinsonNet care or to usual care and then followed the patients for six months. The stated goals of the authors were "(a) to evaluate the implementation of this change in the healthcare system; (b) to record the consequences of implementing ParkinsonNet care, by measuring the health benefits for patients; and (c) to evaluate the influence on societal costs of this new organization of care." Although the primary endpoint (a Patient Specific Index PSI-PD) did not differ between groups, the ParkinsonNet provided an overall greater quality of care while reducing the overall gross financial burden to society[98, 99, 100, 101].

Physical therapy is the most popular and widely utilized form of allied healthcare for Parkinson's-related motor and mobility issues. In fact, the number of published PD physiotherapy and exercise trials has increased by more than 500 percent in recent years. Exciting findings from exercise-based animal studies have revealed the possibility of neuroplastic changes and even the possibility of disease modifying effects. Several clinical trials have suggested that physiotherapy may significantly enhance both motor performance and quality of life. Unfortunately, these findings have to date failed to penetrate into community-based practice, and we will need more studies to convince and to guide the field on how to make exercise programs an international reality.

Today, in Parkinson's disease practices all over the world, exercise is being prescribed more frequently. The evidence trail seems to be pointing toward beneficial effects, but more studies are needed. Hopefully these studies will reveal 1) what kind of exercise is necessary, 2) at what intensity level, and 3) at what frequency the best results will be achieved. Although many practitioners believe that prescribing exercise earlier in the course of Parkinson's disease may yield disease-modifying or neuroprotective benefits, this idea remains unproven. Exercise seems to offer the possibility of both motor and non-motor benefits as well as general health benefits. It is therefore reasonable to consider a daily exercise program, but remember, if you don't break a sweat it probably doesn't count!

❧ Secret No. 7: Exercise Improves Brain Function

CHAPTER 8:

Be Prepared for Hospitalization

"I have a favorite cemetery I go to, because it's really clean and the doctors and nurses are all very nice."

— Jarod Kintz

SEVERAL YEARS AGO WE BECAME alarmed at the number of reports we were receiving from patients regarding negative experiences in the hospital. We decided to investigate these issues by utilizing the international network of National Parkinson Foundation Centers of Excellence. What we discovered from this effort was startling.

Hospitalization in Parkinson's Disease

Our group published a series of three papers that aimed to identify and suggest improvements in care for the hospitalized Parkinson's disease patient. In the first paper, we aimed to review the literature and identify practice gaps in the management of the hospitalized Parkinson's disease patient[102]. We were interested in this general question of hospitalization as many experts had cited that patients with Parkinson's disease were typically admitted to hospitals at higher rates and frequently had longer hospital stays when compared to the general population. Our working group reviewed publications drawn from the previous 40 years. Most papers cited motor disturbances to be a causal factor in the higher rates of admissions and complications[103, 104].

However, other conditions were commonly recorded as the primary reason for hospitalization. These included motor complications, reduced mobility, lack of compliance, inappropriate use of neuroleptics (dopamine blocking drugs), falls, fractures, pneumonia, and other serious medical problems. There were many relevant issues identified and many were preventable or could be improved. Medications, dosages, and specific dosage schedules were critical elements to the success of Parkinson's disease patients in the hospital, but it was unclear if hospital staff members were aware of this issue.

Staff training regarding medications and medication management was lacking, and there was little in the literature suggesting that early mobility and prevention of aspiration pneumonia were critical, despite the fact that it was the number one killer in Parkinson's disease. We concluded that educational programs, recommendations, and guidelines were all desperately needed and that these guidelines would likely save lives, provide a cost savings to the healthcare system, and improve outcomes.

The Management of the Hospitalized Patient

In the second paper, we explored current practices and opinions on the management of the Parkinson's disease (PD) patient in the hospital by utilizing our network of 54 National Parkinson Foundation (NPF) Centers worldwide[105]. We had each of our centers complete an online survey regarding hospitalization of Parkinson's disease patients. These centers were among an elite group of care facilities in the world, and 43 of them carried the prestigious and difficult to obtain Center of Excellence designation. Many centers reported grave concern about the quality of Parkinson's disease-specific care that was provided to their patients when hospitalized. The biggest concerns included adherence to the patient's outpatient medication schedule and the lack of understanding and appreciation by hospital staff of the medications that could worsen Parkinson's disease.

Surprisingly, few NPF Centers of Excellence had an existing policy within their primary hospital that facilitated immediate notification of the Parkinson's doctor if their patient was admitted to the hospital.

Shockingly, notification of hospitalization typically was reported to be directly from the patient or a family member. About one third of centers reported not finding out about their patient being hospitalized until a routine clinic visit following discharge. These visits could occur as far out as many months following discharge. Quick access to outpatient care was lacking across most centers. Elective surgery, falls, fractures, infections, and confusion were all identified as common reasons for hospitalization.

We concluded that there was a need for involvement of a Parkinson's disease specialist or at least a neurologist when patients were admitted to the hospital. Education of hospital staff and clinicians regarding the management of Parkinson's disease, complications, and medications to avoid was critical and needed to be addressed. Most importantly, outpatient access needed to be improved in order to prevent unnecessary hospitalizations.

Risk Factors for Hospitalization

In the third and most important paper, we sought to identify risk factors for hospitalization (emergency room (ER) visits or admissions) among Parkinson's disease patients followed in our National Parkinson Foundation Quality Improvement Initiative. The initiative was modeled after a similar effort put together by Gerry O'Connor at the Dartmouth Health Outcomes Center. Gerry had a crazy but practical idea. He would collect one page of data once a year on all cystic fibrosis patients and use the data to benchmark how centers were doing and to promote best practices. Most leading scientists viewed this approach as a waste of time, energy, and money. The registry, however, paid big dividends and based on issues identified across the network of cystic fibrosis centers nationwide, the average age a cystic fibrosis patient now lives is 10 years longer (from approximately 28 to 38 years of age).

Joyce Oberdorf, the CEO of the National Parkinson Foundation, hired Gerry O'Connor to replicate the same program but to work with our experts to bring the idea to Parkinson's disease. Joyce hired a young talent and data whiz from Harvard University and Cornell University named Peter Schmidt. Peter was hungry to help people after a successful career as an investment banker. Peter, along with Andy Siderowf from the University of Pennsylvania, Mark Guttman from Markham in Toronto, and John Nutt from the University of Oregon, helped to organize a group of skeptical clinician-scientists into the National Parkinson Foundation Quality Improvement Study[77].

The initial data from the initiative yielded 3,060 patients, and shockingly 1,016 (33 percent) had a hospitalization in the first year. Of those, 49 percent had a readmission in the second year. Those who were not hospitalized the first year of the study had a 25 percent risk of a new hospitalization in the second year.

The data from the study was assembled by our young Australian fellow, Anhar Hassan who is now at the Mayo Clinic in Rochester, Minnesota. The surprising wake up call was that PD patients had very high rates of hospitalization (ER visits or admissions) and that these hospitalizations were associated with advanced disease, more co-morbid conditions (e.g. hypertension, heart disease, lung issues, etc.), and a longer time to rise from a chair, walk 10 meters and return to the chair (referred to as a timed up and go test). Quality of life was worse for those hospitalized, and not surprisingly, there was a higher burden on the caregiver. Just as in O'Connor's study of cystic fibrosis, some centers performed better than others suggesting that there may be better ways to improve care and to prevent hospitalization.

Drugs to Avoid in Parkinson's Disease

When in or out of the hospital it is important to understand what drugs should be avoided in Parkinson's disease patients. A good friend of mine and very experienced senior neurologist Ed Steinmetz from Ft. Meyers, Florida, pointed out to me a list of such drugs recently published in the Public Citizen newsletter. The approach was to list every drug associated with a single confirmed or unconfirmed symptom of Parkinson's disease or Parkinsonism. Patients and family members confronted with a simple "drug list" approach may falsely conclude that most medicines are bad for Parkinson's disease and even worse that any medicine may cause Parkinsonism. This concept is, in general, incorrect. Although the approach is well-meaning, it is in need of a major revision as Parkinson's disease is too complex to summarize by simple lists.

It is well known that drugs that block dopamine worsen Parkinson's disease, whereas dopamine replacement therapy (carbidopa/levodopa, Sinemet, dopamine agonists) may improve symptoms. One of the big issues facing many Parkinson's disease patients is psychosis (hallucinations, illusions, and behavioral changes such as paranoia). How does one concomitantly administer dopamine replacement therapy, which may in some cases induce psychosis, while at the same time administer dopamine blocker drugs aimed at alleviating psychosis? Will the drugs cancel each other out?

There are two dopamine blockers that will in general not cancel out dopamine replacement, therefore not appreciably worsen Parkinson's disease. One is Quetiapine (Seroquel) and the other is Clozapine (Clozaril). Clozapine is the more powerful of the two drugs, but it requires weekly blood monitoring. Other classical dopamine blocking drugs, also referred to as neuroleptics (e.g. Haldol), worsen Parkinson's disease. Every Parkinson's disease patient and doctor should be aware of these two drugs that are the preferred treatment for psychosis occurring inside or outside of the hospital.

Patients may not be aware that some common drugs used for conditions such as headache or gastrointestinal dysmotility may also block dopamine and concomitantly worsen Parkinson's disease or alternatively result in Parkinsonism (Parkinson's-like symptoms). These drugs include Prochlorperazine (Compazine), Promethazine (Phenergan), and Metoclopramide (Reglan). These drugs should be avoided. Also, drugs that deplete dopamine such as reserpine and tetrabenazine may worsen Parkinson's disease and should be avoided in most cases. Substitute drugs that do not result in worsening can be utilized, and these include Ondansetron (Zofran) for nausea and erythromycin or domperidone for gastrointestinal motility. Domperidone is not available in the U.S. but can be compounded by specialty pharmacies upon request.

Antidepressants, anxiolytics, mood stabilizers, thyroid replacement drugs, and antihypertensives are in general safe and do not worsen Parkinson's disease. They appear commonly on lists, including those provided by the Public Citizen, but don't be misled. Occasionally, there are reactions that lead to worsening of Parkinson's disease, but these are very rare occurrences. The bigger issue is drug-drug interactions. The most commonly encountered drug-drug interaction in Parkinson's disease is mixing a MAO-B Inhibitor (Selegline, Rasagiline, Azilect, Zelapar, Selegiline Hydrochloride dissolvable) with a pain medicine such as Meperidine (Demerol).

Also, MAO-A Inhibitors (e.g. Pirlindole) should not be taken with antidepressants. It should be kept in mind that in rare instances mixing an antidepressant with another class of drugs can in select cases result in a serotonin syndrome (increased heart rate, tremor, sweating, big pupils, twitchy muscles and hyperactive reflexes.) MAO-B's, in almost all cases, are safe to take concomitantly with antidepressants, though many pharmacists will question the potential interaction and refuse to fill prescriptions. This refusal should be questioned by your doctor.

The list approach to the worst pills in Parkinson's disease and Parkinsonism needs a critical reappraisal. A more refined approach would take into consideration the complexities of Parkinson's disease and would appreciate that with physician guidance and with few exceptions, most drugs can be safely and effectively administered in Parkinson's disease and Parkinsonism. This is inclusive of many of the over the counter pills marked "not for use in Parkinson's disease.[19]"

Aware in Care Campaign

NPF used the information on hospitalization and worst drugs in Parkinson's disease to fuel an effort to assist hospitalized patients. The problem NPF encountered was that patients could not depend on every hospital and every hospital employee worldwide to understand what to do and what not to do in Parkinson's disease management. The idea was to create a kit much like the bag that is packed and ready for a last trimester pregnant woman. The kit that has everything you need to survive the hospitalization.

The kit is large enough to pack your medications and also includes several critical elements:

1. A hospital action plan that provides?tips on how to prepare for the next hospital visit

2. A Parkinson's disease identification bracelet?

3. A medical alert card?

4. A medication form to keep a list of active medications

5. A Parkinson's disease fact sheet?to hand to the hospital staff and to be placed in your chart

6. "I have Parkinson's disease" reminder slips to educate hospital staff

7. A thank you card?for the staff member who provided the highest quality Parkinson's care

The kit reinforces the simple platform that Parkinson's disease patients require their medications on time every time and that many common drugs used in the hospital will worsen Parkinson's disease.

Secrets that can make your hospital stays shorter and potentially improve your condition include:

- Preventable errors in the hospital save lives.

- You and our family should assume the role of the "advocate."

- You and your family must educate all staff and physicians you contact.

- You will need to re-emphasize that Parkinson's disease patients require medications on time every time.

- You will need to educate that Parkinson's disease symptoms worsen with sleep deprivation, stress, infections, and anesthesia/ surgery.

- Be prepared for unplanned hospitalizations, as the percentages predict that they will happen sooner or later with Parkinson's disease.

❧ Secret No. 8- Be Prepared for Hospitalization

CHAPTER 9:

Always Ask About New Therapies

'There's no need for fiction in medicine,' remarks Foster... 'for the facts will always beat anything you fancy.'

— Sir Arthur Conan Doyle

THE FIRST QUESTION A PATIENT asks in the office is about his or her symptoms, but the last and most heartfelt is about the research. "Doc, where is the research going?"

Parkinson's disease research has recently exploded with literally thousands of leading researchers all over the globe. They are all following exciting new leads. In the last two decades alone we have learned more about Parkinson's disease than in the intervening period between the first essay description in 1817 and the introduction of dopamine replacement therapy. We now understand that Parkinson's is not one disease. Parkinson's is actually a syndrome composed of a cluster of similar clinical manifestations such as tremor, shuffling feet, and small handwriting; and that these symptoms occur in a large group of patients who present to their doctors for diagnosis and management. The syndrome is complex and has multiple causes.

The first objective in focusing the research will be to better understand and separate these causes. Important to this effort will be dissecting the changes that occur at the cellular level (i.e. basic science), in the tissues (i.e. pathology, proteins and how they are processed), in the brain circuits (i.e. physiology), and in the DNA (i.e. genetics). Changes in each of these areas will be important to unlocking the Parkinson's disease mystery.

Once we better understand what ignites Parkinson's disease, we can identify potential targets and treatment approaches. Targets for therapy could include a malfunctioning cell or group of cells, a gene, a protein, a protein accumulation, or we could even aim to resurface of an entire neural circuit. Each treatment approach should deliver a therapy aimed at directly addressing the fundamental and underlying problems leading to Parkinson's disease and its consequent symptoms.

One common misconception among Parkinson's disease patients is that symptomatic treatments, disease modifying therapies, and cures are all the same. Each approach has important fundamental differences, and each should be separated. A symptomatic treatment addresses a disease manifestation (e.g. dopamine replacement or deep brain stimulation to treat tremor, rigidity, or slowness). A disease modifying treatment would target slowing of the progression of Parkinson's disease. In contrast, a cure would lead to eradication of disease. Currently we have many medical, surgical, and behavioral symptomatic treatments but no disease modifying therapies and no cures[19]. This reality begs the question, what will it take to get us on the road to a cure?

The Genetic Approach

We have come a long way since James Watson and Francis Crick discovered the double helix structure of DNA in 1953. Genetics and genetic testing have become widely available, and there has been a race to identify all of the possible Parkinson's disease genes. We have confirmed that in five to 10 percent of those diagnosed with Parkinson's disease there will be an identifiable abnormality within their DNA. These alterations in the genetic code, in most cases, can be confirmed by a simple blood test. The current DNA abnormalities are what we have uncovered today. However, there may be many more genetic mutations discovered in the near future. Genetics have provided important clues to the potential underlying causes of Parkinson's disease.

For example, a mutation in the gene that codes for the protein alpha synuclein (SNCA) will lead to a specific form of Parkinson's disease. This observation proved vital to the field and has implications beyond the genetic forms of Parkinson's disease. Accumulation of this protein in the brain has been consistently observed across all cases of Parkinson's disease, therefore the ability to trace it back to a single gene defect has been a critical discovery. There have been other genes such as PARKIN, LRRK2, and PINK1 that all have been linked to the development of Parkinson's disease, and all of these genes have pointed scientists toward possible mechanisms underpinning the disease and also to potential drug targets.

Sergey Brin, one of the co-founders of the internet giant Google, changed the world of Parkinson's disease genetics in a profound way. Now, you might say how in the world did a young computer programmer change the entire field of neurogenetics and genetic testing for a generation of patients? The story as it turns out, is very personal. After a visit to the University of Maryland, Brin discovered that his mother Eugenia had Parkinson's disease. Following this revelation, Brin himself underwent genetic testing. His blood revealed a small mutation in the genetic code known as the LRRK2 mutation. LRRK2 is currently the most commonly known genetic form of Parkinson's disease. Following his own genetic testing, Brin has been famously quoted as saying that he regards his own genetic code to be no different than a computer code. If it is flawed, we just need to fix it. Brin and his wife started a company called 23andme, and this company has offered large-scale genetic testing for Parkinson's disease but without genetic counseling. Genetic counseling is typically provided by trained professionals who explain to patients and families the implications on one's life of unmasking an underlying genetic mutation. Would you live your life differently if you knew you were destined to suffer from a devastating disease?

The lack of genetic counseling from the 23andme company set off a global controversy. The need for it can be illustrated by an important anecdote from another neurological disease, Huntington's, and a pair of sisters named the Wexlers. The Wexler story began when their father was diagnosed with Huntington's disease. Along with Woody Guthrie's family, they started a movement in the late 1960s to raise money for research. This movement yielded the founding of the Hereditary Disease Foundation. Through Wexler funding and the services of multiple scientists from around the globe, the gene for Huntington's disease was identified in 1984 by James Gusella, a researcher based at Massachusetts General Hospital.

The way Huntington's disease works is if you have one parent with the problem, your disease risk is 50 percent, or a one in two chance. These statistics reflect what is known as autosomal dominant inheritance. In autosomal dominant disorders you only need to inherit one copy of an abnormal gene to get a disease. Because the sisters were at risk, and because the gene had been uncovered, the two women had to decide whether or not to be tested.

Most people assume that with the availability of a genetic test, 100 percent of a population would opt for testing. In reality, once patients and families sit down with a genetic counselor and review the implications of unmasking their gene status, approximately 50 percent of patients will make a conscious decision to not be tested. So what did the sisters decide? Alice, the historian from the University of California, was tested and was discovered to be gene negative. Nancy, the Huntington's disease researcher, has yet to be tested. Ironically, Nancy was, and remains, a critical part of the research team involved in the Huntington's disease gene discovery and genetic research both in the United States and in Maracaibo, Venezuela. Nancy has spent the better part of the last 30 years leading trips to Maracaibo to study the largest population of Huntington's disease patients in the world[106]. It was one of the thrills of my career to accompany her and Anne Young, chairperson of the Department of Neurology at Massachusetts General Hospital, on one of these visits.

What has emerged in Parkinson's disease research has been two schools of thought as to how to approach the "cure." The Google approach has been a quantity and data-driven methodology focused on the genetics. Brin and colleagues believe that if they collect enough DNA and enough information on Parkinson's disease sufferers, the problems and solutions will naturally emerge.

This philosophy is in striking contrast to the traditional Parkinson's disease research approach that has been based on the scientific method. Ask important questions and formulate testable hypotheses. Test the hypotheses, and keep the momentum by moving forward with more questions and more hypotheses. The advantage to the scientific method is that it is more direct and more focused. Only time will tell which approach will win the day for Parkinson's disease, and it is possible that both will be important in shaping the new research horizons.

As more and more Parkinson's disease patients and family members receive genetic screening, further improvements in technology continue to be made. One very interesting development has been the X Prize Foundation's $10 million Archin X prize for genomics that was to be awarded to the first team that could build a device and use it to sequence 100 human genomes within 10 days or less. The prize remains unclaimed, however, full genome sequencing is now possible, and costs and techniques continue to be refined. Affluent patients can now pay to have a copy of their complete genetic code generated. So, to add to the ethical discussion of whether or not to be tested for Parkinson's disease, now you must consider whether you want your DNA screened for all known diseases.

There is a complicated twist to this story. Just because you have a gene does not mean you will get a disease. The field of modern genetics is much more complex than Gregor Mendel imagined in the 1850s when he was crossing and making hybrid pea plants. A person can actually have a gene but not develop a disease. This mind-blowing phenomenon means that having a gene defect imparts a risk that is actually variable and less than 100 percent. The future of genetics will need to include information on what potential environmental triggers can turn your DNA on and off. Judith Stern from the University of California has coined the phrase, "the genes load the gun, and the environment pulls the trigger." In Parkinson's disease, there is now a race to identify environmental triggers that can turn your native DNA on and off.

So, let's hypothetically imagine that we wanted to cure the most common genetic form of Parkinson's disease, the LRRK2 or leucine rich repeat kinase type 2 mutation. This gene encodes a protein called dardarin. Dardarin is the Basque word for tremor, although ironically not all Parkinson patients with LRRK2 actually have tremor. People with the LRRK2 mutation in their DNA have an increased risk for both Parkinson's disease and Crohn's disease, a gastrointestinal disorder. Mutations in LRRK2 are thought to lead to a loss of function in your body's cells and eventually to cell death. Therefore, any cure approach would have to address stopping cell death.

There are several promising approaches to stopping LRRK2-related cell death in the brain. These approaches have included a direct gene therapy paradigm (e.g. inserting healthy LRRK2 cells), targeting LRRK2 or its protein products through drugs or trophic factors, or alternatively targeting some downstream effect of LRRK2 to hopefully prevent brain cell death. Because LRRK2 is a "loss of function" gene, some investigators believe it would be more amenable to gene therapy as opposed to another Parkinson's gene, the PARKIN mutation, which leads to a "gain of function" within cells of the body.

The Genes Load the Gun and the Environment Pulls the Trigger

Pesticides, Agent Orange, and potential environmental risk factors for the development of Parkinson's disease continue to make the news. Patients and families may be confronted by worrisome headlines on chemicals and Parkinson's disease, to most of which they may never be exposed.

Drs. Samuel Goldman and Carly Tanner from the Sunnyvale Parkinson's Institute studied twins from a WWII Veterans Cohort. By utilizing twin pairs (half were identical twins), researchers limited the potential effects of genetics on the development of Parkinson's disease. One person from each twin pair was required to have been diagnosed with Parkinson's disease. A very careful occupational and hobby history was then extracted. First hand histories from patients were sparse with spouses and siblings providing secondhand proxy histories in most cases. An occupational hygienist was used to help determine exposure. An occupational hygienist is a carefully trained professional who can independently determine exposures, hazards, or risks in a workplace environment. The hygienist along with the researchers examined six solvents and determined that only trichloroethylene (TCE) was associated with an increased risk (6.1 times) of developing Parkinson's disease in men. Additionally, men exposed to TCE or to another chemical called PERC (tetrachloroethylene) had an 8.9 times increased risk of developing Parkinson's disease.

Interestingly n-hexane, xylene, and toluene, which have all been thought to be potentially associated with the development of Parkinson's disease, did not show an increased risk in this cohort. All of the studies of environmental exposures should be interpreted with caution, and patients and families should look for common themes among multiple research reports as there is potential for error in these types of population-based studies[107, 108, 109].

An important question a patient or family member should ask about TCE is what kind of work might lead to an exposure. The following is a list of potential items that might put one in contact with TCE:

- Grease remover

- Typewriter correction fluid

- Paints and strippers

- Carpet cleaners and spot removers

- Adhesives

- Computer part cleaners

- Decaffeinated coffees

- Dry cleaning

- Textile plants

- Anaesthetics in an operating room setting

The following is a list of the highest risk occupations associated with TCE exposure:

- Electricians

- Dry cleaners

- Industrial machinists and repair crews

- Health care workers

Patients and families should appreciate that there is a difference between acute TCE exposure and chronic TCE exposure. Acute, high dose exposure seems to depress the central nervous system and may lead to breathing problems, heart arrhythmias, coma, and a host of other problems. Acute TCE may also prove to be a nasty skin irritant. When we talk about TCE exposure and Parkinson's disease, we are referring to chronic long-term exposure. Chronic exposure has also been associated with unsteadiness, dizziness, headaches, memory loss, and many other symptoms. The current study by Samuel Goldman suggests that Parkinson's disease risk may need to be added to the potential sequelae of chronic TCE exposure.

Patients and families should also be aware that the risk factors for Parkinson's disease may be inclusive of many environmental exposures and not just TCE. Dana Hancock and colleagues at Duke

University recently reported that insecticides and herbicides, especially organochlorines and organophosphorus compounds, increased the risk of Parkinson's disease even in those without a family history. Pesticides and environmental risk factors therefore have emerged as important considerations in the development of Parkinson's disease[110, 111]. Patients, families and physicians should all be aware of these chemicals and should assess their risks for exposure[19].

One of the most important and emerging areas of research has been the interaction between genes and the environment. Some researchers call this area epigenetics. It is becoming clear that just because you have a gene does not mean you will develop a disease. Similarly, just because you have an environmental exposure it does not mean you will get Parkinson's disease. Most scientists believe there is likely a two-hit hypothesis at work. In other words, it likely takes more than one event to precipitate Parkinson's disease. So indeed, the genes may load the gun, and the environment or another unknown factor may pull the trigger.

Stem Cell Approach

A breakthrough scientific development in the past year has been the ability of scientists to manipulate skin cells to be reprogrammed to become what is known as pluripotent stem cells. Pluripotent means that the cells, once generated, gain the ability to form multiple different cell types in the body. How do scientists pull off this remarkable accomplishment? In their laboratories, scientists induce the expression of several transcription factors that encode the genetic maps in any individual person. By inducing these factors, they can generate what has been referred to as induced pluripotent stem cells or iPS stem cell.

In the initial experiments, a combination of the chemicals Oct4, Sox2, Klf4, and Myc were used to induce a transition of fibroblasts (skin cells) into stable and self-renewing cells. Remarkably, these cells very closely resemble embryonic stem cells. The ability to generate stem cells from skin cells should largely end the debates surrounding the use of human embryos for stem cell research, as human embryos will rarely be required.

The reprogramming of stem cells has now been demonstrated in a wide range of cell types, and it reaches far beyond skin cells. Several newer techniques have been employed to reprogram cells from various body tissues. These methods have included nuclear transfer, cell fusion, explantation of cells in culture, and the transduction of cells with several well-defined factors and chemicals. The exact molecular mechanism underpinning the reprogramming remains uncertain, but it is important to appreciate the critical discovery that scientists can reproducibly generate stem cells from many sources, and they can reprogram them into many cell types.

iPS stem cells have raised the possibility and the hope of curing Parkinson's disease for patients and family members living on all continents. Could it be possible through this cell reprogramming technique to generate tailor made cells and use them as neurotherapeutics? Recent rat and primate studies have revealed that these cells can be manufactured and transplanted, then survive and help the symptoms of Parkinson's disease. So why then have we fallen short of a cure with stem cells?

There are major hurdles that must be crossed to move to the clinical implementation of therapeutic preparations of iPS stem cells. It is critical that these preparations be completely pure and free of undifferentiated cells that may have the future potential to form tumors. The most significant challenge will be the development of techniques to facilitate the precise delivery of iPS cells into patients and the functional engraftment of these cells into the appropriate and complex Parkinson's circuitry. Scientists are now beginning to appreciate that the basal ganglia brain motor and non-motor circuits are so elaborate and so multiplexed that simply transplanting cells into one or more spots will not be enough for the cure.

There are, however, several direct and immediate applications of iPS cells to Parkinson's disease research. Drug screening and disease modeling will be two potential and immediate uses for the technology.

Improvements in high throughput drug screening using iPS cells may allow identification of compounds that could be used as drugs to treat the symptoms of Parkinson's disease.

A Targeted Viral Approach

A common question asked by Parkinson's disease patients is "what is gene therapy?" Gene therapy is placing genetic information (DNA) into the cells and tissues of humans with Parkinson's disease. In the purest form, a defective part of the genome is replaced with a new copy. The most interesting part of the evolving story of gene therapy has been the use of a virus as a vector to carry genetic information into the brain. Viruses can be deactivated and safely used for this purpose, and they can be tagged with either genetic material or neurotrophins. Neurotrophins are a family of proteins that induce survival, development, and proper functioning of brain cells.

There have been three major gene therapy or neurotrophin trials in humans with Parkinson's disease. The first trial aimed to deliver amino acid decarboxylase and was sponsored by a company called Avigen. A brain enzyme, amino acid decarboxylase, enhances the effectiveness of dopaminergic replacement medicines such as levodopa (Sinemet or Madopar). This therapy was aimed at improving motor symptoms, reducing medication dosages, and reducing side effects. In the first study, there was some mild improvement noted, but the therapy fell short of its anticipated potential. It did, however, prove to be safe[112].

The second major trial delivered neurturin, a protein that may repair and rescue dopamine cells in the brain[113]. The company Ceregene provided the neurturin. Neuturin belongs to the same protein family as glial cell derived neurotrophic factor (GDNF), which was another gene therapy that had disappointing results in a recently publicized Parkinson's disease trial sponsored by Amgen. The neurturin trial, like the GDNF trial, was negative, but the investigators are currently repeating the study as they believe they inserted the neurotrophin into a suboptimal location.

The final gene therapy trial focused on an enzyme called glutamic acid decarboxylase (GAD) and was sponsored by Neurologix. Michael Kaplitt, Matt During, and colleagues from Cornell University reported in the Lancet in 2007 the "Safety and tolerability of gene therapy with an adeno-associated virus (AAV) borne GAD gene for Parkinson's disease: an open label, phase I trial."

The subthalamic nucleus (STN) is a brain structure that spews a chemical called glutamate onto another structure in the brain called the globus pallidus. Many treatment schemes have focused on controlling or neuromodulating the output from this STN region. One such approach has been inserting a lead into the brain and introducing electricity in order to change the firing pattern emanating from the STN (deep brain stimulation). Kaplitt and colleagues developed an alternative and innovative approach by using gene therapy to change the STN from a chemically excitatory nucleus to a chemically inhibitory one.

What they proposed and pulled off was very clever. They measured the safety, tolerability, and preliminary effectiveness of the "transfer of the glutamic acid decarboxylase (GAD) gene with adeno-associated virus (AAV) into the STN of patients with Parkinson's disease." The original study had only 11 patients, and the group was similar to those typically chosen to undergo deep brain stimulation (under 70 years old with on-off medication related Parkinson's fluctuations and only minimal cognitive dysfunction). The most important outcome was that there were no adverse events related to the gene therapy. Significant improvements in the motor scores of the patients were also seen, but the results were not of the magnitude that would be required to rock the field.

The amount of change in the motor scores was similar to what has been observed following deep brain stimulation, although longer-term follow-up will be needed. Many experts believe that gene therapy has a high "bar" to pass, as the results of deep brain stimulation have provided excellent benefits in a similar group of patients. Preliminary analyses point to the benefit (similar to deep brain stimulation) as being predominantly in motor function and not in areas of non-motor or levodopa resistant symptoms (depression, sleep, gait, balance, communication, etc.). No one knows if changing the excitatory function of the nucleus into an inhibitory function will affect learning, but this is a point that will require close follow up[114, 115, 116].

The most important finding of the Kaplitt study was that gene therapy was successfully used in humans with Parkinson's disease and that the success will hopefully open the door to future gene therapies as well as combination therapies (genes plus stem cells, genes plus medications, or genes plus deep brain stimulation).

The three published gene and trophic factor viral therapy approaches were all clever ways to address the disabling symptoms in Parkinson's disease. What will it take though for gene therapy to deliver a cure? Ultimately, we need to better understand the target and type of patient we will need to treat with this approach. We will need a target that if modified will arrest the progression of Parkinson's disease, and we will need to deliver the gene and/or trophic factor early enough in the disease to make a difference for the patient.

Small Interfering RNA Approach

Small interfering ribonucleic acid (RNA), also known as siRNA, is a class of double stranded RNA molecules that can interfere or promote expression of a particular gene. The interference technique can be used to determine the function of a particular gene and also to develop targets for drug therapy. Your body's genetic code is made up of four nucleotides (molecules that make up your DNA and RNA): adenine, guanine, cytosine, and thymine. These four nucleotides are carefully ordered, and they are transcribed into something called RNA. RNA is then transcribed or read to make the body's proteins. The technology of siRNA was designed as a way to use double strands of RNA to alter the expression of your DNA.

The siRNA technique was first described in London by David Baulcombe's laboratory, which was focused at the time on gene splicing in plants. Baulcombe had no idea how important this technique would become. Later, Thomas Tuschl published a paper in the journal Nature introducing the technique to mammals, and instantly with this single publication, the field acquired a promising new therapeutic tool. Today, there is great hope that this technique can be applied across many diseases. There have been recent attempts at using siRNA to treat macular degeneration, Ebola virus, and other diseases. To date, however, the technology has not proven to be a robust one within human conditions, and issues have arisen such as immune responses (e.g. your body attacking itself) that can be accidentally set off by the introduction of siRNA.

Interestingly, in macular degeneration the siRNAs were designed to knock down the gene important to blood vessel growth also known as angiogenesis. Researchers found that the siRNAs were effective, not because of a direct effect against the gene, but rather due to the body's own immune response. Future trials will need to take this factor into consideration.

In Ebola, preliminary findings have been more dramatic and much more promising. Researchers from Boston University believe they have uncovered a technique using siRNA that may prove to be the first treatment for this devastating virus. Preliminary trials on primates have been promising, and it will be interesting to see how siRNA works when applied to the next Ebola outbreak[117, 118, 119].

Converting siRNA into a therapy for Parkinson's disease has, however, proven to be challenging. When siRNA was used to target the gene that leads to alpha-synuclein overexpression in Parkinson's disease, it did not have the expected robust and positive effects. siRNA has baffled Parkinson's disease researchers in critical areas such as the best way to deliver the therapy, at what target to aim, and the unexpected and unanticipated off-target side effects. (Off target refers to unintended consequences on other cells and tissues.) If researchers can devise better ways to harness siRNA therapy, it could prove a very powerful symptomatic treatment or even a cure for some of the genetic forms of Parkinson's disease.

The Optogenetic Approach

Francis Crick, one of the most famous scientists of our generation, described a double helix structure that is now known to characterize human DNA. (He published this discovery in 1953 with his colleague James Watson.) In the 1970s, Crick discussed in Scientific American, a wish list for future discoveries, including the use of light to control human cells. Light science and light therapy have since been considered both "crazy and far-fetched." However, recent discoveries in the early 21st century have dramatically changed this point of view. Thanks to some very clever scientists, a new field called optogenetics was born, and in the past year it has developed into one of the most important areas in Parkinson's and also in science.

What is optogenetics? "Opto" refers to placing light onto the brain to activate channels and/or enzymes that will ultimately change brain cell firing. The technique is specific and has the potential to add or to delete firing patterns from the brain's native cells. Additionally, brain cell firing can be manipulated at precise millisecond intervals. The fiber-optic light source can be mounted on the skull or placed deep within the brain.

The genetics part of optogenetics utilizes a simple virus carrier system to deliver genes to the brain. The most important of these genetic deliveries has been opsin, which is one of the structures that can be turned on by the light. The most important known opsin used for this technology is Channelrhodopsin-2. This opsin was derived by scientists from algae-based systems. By shining light onto the inserted genetic alteration (opsin), scientists can probe the brain's inner conversations (firing of cells). The technique has allowed investigators to move past the classical genetic animal manipulations and models and obtain greater specificity in their experiments.

Alexxai Kravitz and colleagues from the pioneering optogenetics group at Stanford University published an important paper about Parkinson's disease in Nature Medicine[120]. The authors were able to demonstrate that optogenetics could either worsen or alternatively improve an animal model of Parkinsonism. The investigators performed a simple experiment where they manipulated the well-established basal ganglia direct and indirect pathways, which are well known suspects implicated in the genesis of Parkinson's disease. The authors reported:

"optogenetic control of direct- and indirect-pathway cells in medium spiny projection neurons, achieved through a viral expression of channelrhodopsin-2 in mice. Excitation of the indirect-pathway medium spiny neurons elicited a parkinsonian state, distinguished by increased freezing, bradykinesia and decreased locomotor initiations. Activation of direct-pathway medium spiny neurons reduced freezing and increased locomotion."

A month prior to this Nature paper, Bass and colleagues from Wake Forest University described an optogenetic approach to controlling dopamine release[121]. Since these publications, scores of work in Parkinson's disease has appeared.

Activating brain circuits by using both light and genetics has thus evolved from a science fiction dream into a reality. The technique will likely be refined over the next decade, and it will have tremendous potential to unlock important clues underlying the disease processes ultimately responsible for Parkinson's disease. Optogenetics may also open novel therapeutic possibilities. The technology will help us shine a light on this common and often disabling human neurodegenerative condition, but whether it can be harnessed or combined with stem cells or other therapies to move us toward a cure remains unknown. It is likely we will in the near future observe channelrhodopsin-2 inserted into target specific cell types in the Parkinson's brain, hopefully as a powerful symptomatic therapy. It is also likely that the founder of optogenetics, Karl Deisseroth, will one day receive the Nobel Prize.

Targeting Proteins and Protein Degradation Pathways

Scientists have referred to the pathways leading to Parkinson's disease collectively as a neurodegenerative cascade. In very simple terms, the brain must process proteins in order to perform everyday functions. During the degenerative cascade, proteins are tagged with a substance called ubiquitin, and they are directed to the brain's trash compactors called proteosomes. During the process, proteins can misfold and also aggregate or pile up. Some leading researchers believe that one potential cure strategy would be to simply target the neurodegenerative cascade and alter it before the misfolding and aggregation set in. Several compounds and gene therapy approaches are currently in development to tackle this issue.

A High-Content Drug Screening Approach

The advances in understanding the cells and genetics underlying Parkinson's disease have made high throughput drug screening a reality. The way this technique works is surprisingly simple. A researcher identifies a particular cell, protein, gene, or element of interest. A microtiter plate is then used. These plates have thousands of little divets in them called wells, and the wells can be filled with an element chosen by the Parkinson's researcher. A robot can then apply libraries of potential drugs or therapeutic agents to each well. Many of these applied drugs are already FDA approved for other uses, therefore could be immediately used on patients. The researcher then looks through the wells searching for a "hit" or an indication of an anticipated positive reaction to the combination. High-throughput drug screening using modern automated systems should make the task of searching for Parkinson's disease drugs faster and more efficient.

There are problems with this approach though. First, just because a hit is identified does not mean that it will translate into a safe and effective therapy for Parkinson's disease patients. Second, to test each Parkinson's drug in clinical trials requires thousands of patients and tens of millions of dollars. Finally, each hit may have specificity to certain genetic or other forms of Parkinson's disease, and it is possible that it will not be widely applicable to everyone with Parkinson's symptoms. One major challenge for high-throughput screening will be the advent of an efficient pipeline system that will bring relevant and high potential Parkinson's drugs to market faster.

Neuroprotection Exploratory Trials in Parkinson's Disease

Neuroprotection Exploratory Trials in Parkinson's Disease (NET-PD) was a concept introduced many years ago by the National Institutes of Health as a consortium of centers to test promising therapies for Parkinson's disease. My colleague and close friend Ramon Rodriguez, M.D., runs one at the University of Florida, and he taught me how the process works. NET-PD was designed to evaluate pharmacological approaches to slow disease progression. To date, the consortium has endeavored to test Coenzyme Q10, GPi-1485, minocycline, and creatine. Each of these four compounds has had a large quantity of research to support the potential positive benefits in Parkinson's disease.

To date, only creatine remains a possible disease-modifying approach, though studies of creatine remain ongoing and inconclusive. One major criticism of this approach has been that the drugs have been selected by expert consensus, which considers the potential risks, benefits, and also scientific data, although the selections are still overall opinions from leading experts and far from fact. The cost of this approach is substantial with tens of millions of dollars being spent, and the return on investment being small. The field will need to better refine the process of drug development in the Parkinson's disease pipeline so that once a drug reaches the NET-PD or a manufacturer sponsored trial, the odds of success can be improved.

Parkinson's Vaccine

A new therapy for Parkinson's disease has recently entered testing in human patients. The Austrian company AFFiRiS A.G. launched a two-year clinical trial of a vaccine that was designed to stop Parkinson's disease progression.

Parkinson's disease involves a neurodegeneration that is associated with deposition of a brain protein known as alpha-synuclein. This protein clumps and seems to spread throughout the brain as Parkinson's disease progresses. Many experts believe that much of the damage in Parkinson's disease traces to the failure of the brain to process and clear these protein deposits.

The idea underpinning the Parkinson's vaccine is simple. Patients will receive four injections with the hope that they will stimulate an immune system response against alpha-synuclein and that antibodies will be raised and will attack bad brain proteins, ultimately clearing them. Thirty two human Parkinson's disease patients will be part of a two-year safety and tolerability study which has been named the PD01A project. The study is now underway in Vienna, and it aims to modify disease progression in Parkinson's disease.

It is important to keep in mind that not all experts believe that removal of these brain proteins will result in clinically meaningful changes and disease modification. Additionally, we must keep in mind that one highly publicized attempt to remove the Tau protein in Alzheimer's patients led to serious safety concerns and termination of a vaccine study known as AN1792 because several patients developed a serious meningoencephalitis.

What patients need to know about the vaccine is that it is still in the very early stages of testing, but the idea is novel, and the approach is promising. Safety, tolerability, and clinical efficacy will need to be demonstrated before the vaccine can move to the next phase of clinical testing. The hope is that clearing Parkinson's-associated brain proteins will translate into disease modification. A similar approach is also being tested in other diseases such as Alzheimer's disease, diabetes, and atherosclerosis.

New Drugs or Therapies May be Available in Your Clinic

There are many promising approaches to addressing the disabling symptoms of Parkinson's disease. Exciting therapeutic advances have been recently introduced and refined within a few short years. The creativity and resourcefulness of this generation of scientists and clinicians will continue to move us toward new therapies. You may be eligible to receive a new therapy in the setting of a clinical trial. Ask your doctor at every visit what is new, exciting, and promising. Consider whether you would like to be part of a clinical trial and catalyze the critical movement toward better therapies and more creative approaches to combat this disease.

❧ Secret No. 9: Always Ask About New Therapies

CHAPTER 10:

Kindle Hope into Happiness and a Meaningful Life

IHAVE BEEN HONORED TO SHARE in the lives of thousands of Parkinson's disease patients. My path has been well defined through my many interactions with them. Their problems have become my problems. I know that my job is to shelter their worry and concern so they can have the opportunity for a full and meaningful life.

The journey of the Parkinson's disease patient is fueled by hope, and I have come to realize that it is the hope that ultimately leads to their happiness. It is the hope that will continue to define them through the sometimes difficult journey. The general public may confuse Parkinson's disease for Lou Gehrig's or Alzheimer's, but we must remind the Parky that they are very different and on average have an opportunity to live a long and healthy life. Important tips to kindle the hope into happiness include:

- Do not be defined by the disease.

- Possess and grow strong core values.

- Embrace family and friends.

- Develop a vision for who you want to be and live that vision.

- Share the journey with Parkinson's and other chronic disease patients and families.

- Be aware of drugs, timing, and side effects.

- Exercise every day, and be ready for an unplanned hospitalization.

- Choose an empathetic doctor.

- Visit an interdisciplinary team of Parkinson's specialists at least once a year (physical therapy, occupational therapy, psychologist, psychiatrist, speech/swallow therapist, social worker).

- Be aware that making your brain electric may one day be helpful to your disease symptoms.

- Ask frequently about new drugs, surgeries, and behavioral treatments.

- Maximize the symptomatic treatment of your disease, and do not be consumed by the search for a cure.

- Beware those who will try to hijack your hope to make a dollar (glutathione therapy, chelation, fee for stem cell treatment, miracle cures).

Regardless of your religion or your political position, hope is the most powerful weapon you can employ to combat Parkinson's disease.

You may contact the author directly at michaelokunmd@gmail.com as we welcome any comments to make this book or future books better

There is a free patient and family oriented blog with lots of updated Parkinson's treatment tips at the book's website address: http://www.parkinsonsecrets.com

The website also contains biographies of the non-English translators

Glossary of Terms:

BENSERAZIDE/LEVODOPA (MADOPAR)- A FORM OF dopamine replacement used in Europe and other regions
Carbidopa/levodopa (Sinemet)- a form of dopamine replacement used in the United States and other regions

DBS- deep brain stimulation

Dopamine agonists- unlike simple dopamine replacement therapy (Sinemet or Madopar), dopamine agonists tickle the dopamine receptor in the brain. Common dopamine agonists include Pramipexole (Mirapex), Ropinerole (Requip), Cabergoline Dopamine Dysregulation Syndrome- an addiction-like disorder associated with craving and overuse of Sinemet or Madopar (Dostinex), Pergolide (Permax), Rotigotine (Neupro). Rotigotine is a patch formulation.

Monoamine Oxidase B Inhibitors- a drug treatment for Parkinson's disease that works by inhibiting the breakdown of dopamine. Common monoamine oxidase inhibitors include generic Selegiline, Zydis Selegiline dissolvable (Zelapar Zydis), and Azilect (Rasagiline). MAO-B inhibitors when given in low dosage are relatively safe for Parkinson's disease, even when mixed with other medicines. It is MAO-A that is associated with more drug-drug interactions. MAO-A's are rarely used in Parkinson's disease.

Impulse Control Disorders- behavioral issues typically associated with dopamine agonist use (binge eating, gambling, hypersexuality, other inappropriate behaviors)

Lewy Bodies- protein depositions that contain alpha-synuclein. These depositions are the pathological hallmark of Parkinson's disease.

Punding- compulsive behavior in which the sufferer performs repetitive mechanical tasks

Translated versions of this book:

English- Michael S. Okun, M.D.
Portuguese- Mariana Moscovich, M.D.
Spanish- Daniel Martinez, M.D.
Chinese- Yun Peng, M.D.
Japanese- Genko Oyama, M.D., Ph.D.
Filipino- Criscley Go, M.D.
Korean- Ho-Won Lee, M.D.
Arabic- Omar Alsanaidi, M.D.
Swedish- Beata Ferencz, M.Sc.
German- Christine Daniels, M.D.
French- Nadira AitSahlia, M.D.
Urdu- Mustafa Siddiqui, M.D.
Thai- Natlada Limotai, M.D.
Indonesian Bahasa- Frandy Susatia, M.D.
Hindi (Indian)- Shankar Kulkarni, PhD.
Marathi (Indian)- Aparna Shukla, M.D.
Telugu (Indian)- Ashok Sriram, M.D.
Tamil (Indian)- Vinata Vedam-Mai, PhD.
Italian- Marco Sassi, M.D.

Bengali- Maria Hack
Russian- Mindaugas Bazys, M.D.
Dutch- Peggy Spauwen, M.Sc.
Polish- Emila Sitek, M.D., Jaroslaw Slawek, M.D.
Turkish- Zeynep Tüfekcioglu, M.D., Dr.Hasmet A. Hanagasi

About the Author:

Michael S. Okun, M.D., is considered a world's authority on Parkinson's disease treatment, and his publications provide a voice and an outlet to empower people living with this disease worldwide. He is currently Professor, Administrative Director, and Co-director of the University of Florida Center for Movement Disorders and Neurorestoration, part of the Center for Translational Research in Neurodegenerative Diseases, the McKnight Brain Institute, and the University of Florida College of Medicine. The center is unique in that it is has more than 45 interdisciplinary faculty members from diverse areas of campus all of whom are dedicated to care, outreach, education, and research. All specialists are housed in one place, providing a model for a better experience for the Parkinson's disease patient. Dr. Okun has been dedicated to this interdisciplinary care concept for Parkinson's disease, and since his appointment as the National Medical Director for the National Parkinson Foundation in 2006, he has worked with the more than 40 international NPF centers of excellence to help foster the best possible environments for care, research, and outreach in Parkinson disease, dystonia, Tourette, and movement disorders. Dr. Okun was one of the driving forces behind the creation of the Center for Movement Disorders and Neurorestoration and its completely patient-centric approach to care. Dr. Okun has been supported by grants from the National Parkinson Foundation, the National Institutes of Health, the Parkinson Alliance, and the Michael J. Fox Foundation, and he currently runs the online international "Ask The Expert" forums on the National Parkinson Foundation website. The forum is a free service that answers questions from every continent (except Antartica) and has more than 10,000 postings in the last three years alone.

Dr. Okun has dedicated much of his career to the development of care centers for people suffering with movement disorders. He has also has enjoyed a prolific research career exploring non-motor basal ganglia brain features and has participated in pioneering studies exploring the cognitive, behavioral, and mood effects of deep brain stimulation (DBS). Dr. Okun holds the Adelaide Lackner Professorship in Neurology, has published more than 300 peer-reviewed articles and chapters, is a published poet (Lessons From the Bedside, 1995), and has served as a reviewer for more than 25 major medical journals including JAMA and the New England Journal of Medicine. He has been invited to speak about Parkinson's disease and movement disorders all over the world. His published works can be found in many sources and many languages including the New England Journal of Medicine and the patient forums and blogs at the National Parkinson Foundation. Visitors from around the world come to Gainesville, Florida for his opinion on current Parkinson's treatments, and he is a highly sought after international speaker. He has written many popular books including "Ask the Expert" about Parkinson's disease and "Lessons from the Bedside." You can email Dr. Okun directly at okun@neurology.ufl.edu if you have tips or improvements to suggest for this book or future books.

You may also find useful information on three Parkinson's blogs run by Dr. Okun:

http://www.Parkinsonsecrets.com
http://mdc.mbi.ufl.edu/category/treatment/parkinsons-treatment-tips http://www.parkinson.org/Patients/Patients—On-The-Blog.aspx

Selected References

1. Wang, S.-C., Lu Xun, a Biography1984: Foreign Languages Press.

2. Steinbeck, J., Travels with Charley in Search of America. Penguin Classic2012: Penguin.

3. Bhalla, S., Quotes of Gandhi1995: UBS Publishers Distributors.

4. Dorsey, E.R., et al., Projected number of people with Parkinson disease in the most populous nations, 2005 through 2030. Neurology, 2007. 68(5): p. 384-6.

5. Dungy, T., The Mentor Leader: Secrets to Building People and Teams That Win Consistently2010: Tyndale Momentum.

6. From James Parkinson to Friederich Lewy: leaving landmarks for further research journeys. Funct Neurol, 2003. 18(2): p. 63-4.

7. Holdorff, B., Friedrich Heinrich Lewy (1885-1950) and his work. J Hist Neurosci, 2002. 11(1): p. 19-28.

8. Paterniti, M., Driving Mr. Albert: A Trip Across America with Einstein's Brain2001: Dial Press.

9. Abelson, J.N., Simon, M.I., Wetzel, R., Amyloid, Proteins, Prions, and Other Aggregates. Vol. 309. 1999: Academic Press.

10. Braak, E. and H. Braak, Silver staining method for demonstrating Lewy bodies in Parkinson's disease and argyrophilic oligodendrocytes in multiple system atrophy. J Neurosci Methods, 1999. 87(1): p. 111-5.

11. Braak, H. and E. Braak, Pathoanatomy of Parkinson's disease. J Neurol, 2000. 247 Suppl 2: p. II3-10.

12. Braak, H., et al., Pattern of brain destruction in Parkinson's and Alzheimer's diseases. J Neural Transm, 1996. 103(4): p. 455-90.

13. Takahashi, H., [Pathology of neurodegenerative diseases: with special reference to Parkinson's disease and amyotrophic lateral sclerosis]. Rinsho Shinkeigaku, 2002. 42(11): p. 1085-7.

14. Cooper, J.M.J., Woodrow Wilson: A Biography2011: Vintage First Edition.

15. Carp, L., George Gershwin-illustrious American composer: his fatal glioblastoma. Am J Surg Pathol, 1979. 3(5): p. 473-8.

16. Ljunggren, B., The case of George Gershwin. Neurosurgery, 1982. 10(6 Pt 1): p. 733-6.

17. Parent, M. and A. Parent, Substantia nigra and Parkinson's disease: a brief history of their long and intimate relationship. Can J Neurol Sci, 2010. 37(3): p. 313-9.

18. Finger, S., Origins of Neuroscience: A History into Explanations into Brain Function2001: Oxford University Press.

19. Okun, M.S., Fernandez, H.H., Ask the Doctor About Parkinson's Disease2009: Demos Health.

20. Jin, D.Z., N. Fujii, and A.M. Graybiel, Neural representation of time in cortico-basal ganglia circuits. Proc Natl Acad Sci U S A, 2009. 106(45): p. 19156-61.

21. Sacks, O., Awakenings1999: Vintage.

22. Langston, J.W., The Case of the Frozen Addict1996: Vintage.

23. Stegemoller, E.L., T. Simuni, and C. MacKinnon, Effect of movement frequency on repetitive finger movements in patients with Parkinson's disease. Mov Disord, 2009. 24(8): p. 1162-9.

24. Stegemoller, E.L., T. Simuni, and C.D. Mackinnon, The effects of Parkinson's disease and age on syncopated finger movements. Brain Res, 2009. 1290: p. 12-20.

25. Benabid, A.L., [Stimulation therapies for Parkinson's disease: over the past two decades]. Bull Acad Natl Med, 2010. 194(7): p. 1273-86.

26. Benabid, A.L., et al., Long-term electrical inhibition of deep brain targets in movement disorders. Mov Disord, 1998. 13 Suppl 3: p. 119-25.

27. Benabid, A.L., et al., Chronic VIM thalamic stimulation in Parkinson's disease, essential tremor and extra-pyramidal dyskinesias. Acta Neurochir Suppl (Wien), 1993. 58: p. 39-44.

28. Benabid, A.L., J.F. Le Bas, and P. Pollak, [Therapeutic and physiopathological contribution of electric stimulation of deep brain structures in Parkinson's disease]. Bull Acad Natl Med, 2003. 187(2): p. 305-19; discussion 319-22.

29. Benazzouz, A. and M. Hallett, Mechanism of action of deep brain stimulation. Neurology, 2000. 55(12 Suppl 6): p. S13-6.

30. Lozano, A.M., et al., Deep brain stimulation for Parkinson's disease: disrupting the disruption. Lancet Neurol, 2002. 1(4): p. 225-31.

31. Lozano, A.M. and H. Eltahawy, How does DBS work? Suppl Clin Neurophysiol, 2004. 57: p. 733-6.

32. McIntyre, C.C., et al., Uncovering the mechanism(s) of action of deep brain stimulation: activation, inhibition, or both. Clin Neurophysiol, 2004. 115(6): p. 1239-48.

33. McIntyre, C.C., et al., How does deep brain stimulation work? Present understanding and future questions. J Clin Neurophysiol, 2004. 21(1): p. 40-50.

34. Okun, M.S., Deep-brain stimulation for Parkinson's disease. N Engl J Med, 2012. 367(16): p. 1529-38.

35. Lee, K.H., et al., Emerging techniques for elucidating mechanism of action of deep brain stimulation. Conf Proc IEEE Eng Med Biol Soc, 2011. 2011: p. 677-80.

36. Lee, K.H., et al., High frequency stimulation abolishes thalamic network oscillations: an electrophysiological and computational analysis. J Neural Eng, 2011. 8(4): p. 046001.

37. Vedam-Mai, V., et al., Deep brain stimulation and the role of astrocytes. Mol Psychiatry, 2012. 17(2): p. 124-31, 115.

38. Steindler, D.A., M.S. Okun, and B. Scheffler, Stem cell pathologies and neurological disease. Mod Pathol, 2012. 25(2): p. 157-62.

39. Wang, S., et al., Neurogenic potential of progenitor cells isolated from postmortem human Parkinsonian brains. Brain Res, 2012. 1464: p. 61-72.

40. Okun, M.S. and K.D. Foote, Parkinson's disease DBS: what, when, who and why? The time has come to tailor DBS targets. Expert Rev Neurother, 2010. 10(12): p. 1847-57.

41. Oyama, G., et al., Selection of deep brain stimulation candidates in private neurology practices: referral may be simpler than a computerized triage system. Neuromodulation, 2012. 15(3): p. 246-50; discussion 250.

42. Okun, M.S., et al., Development and initial validation of a screening tool for Parkinson disease surgical candidates. Neurology, 2004. 63(1): p. 161-3.

43. Alexander, G.E., M.D. Crutcher, and M.R. DeLong, Basal ganglia-thalamocortical circuits: parallel substrates for motor, oculomotor, "prefrontal" and "limbic" functions. Prog Brain Res, 1990. 85: p. 119-46.

44. Alexander, G.E., M.R. DeLong, and P.L. Strick, Parallel organization of functionally segregated circuits linking basal ganglia and cortex. Annu Rev Neurosci, 1986. 9: p. 357-81.

45. DeLong, M. and T. Wichmann, Deep brain stimulation for movement and other neurologic disorders. Ann N Y Acad Sci, 2012. 1265: p. 1-8.

46. DeLong, M.R., et al., Role of basal ganglia in limb movements. Hum Neurobiol, 1984. 2(4): p. 235-44.

47. Delong, M.R., et al., Functional organization of the basal ganglia: contributions of single-cell recording studies. Ciba Found Symp, 1984. 107: p. 64-82.

48. Goetz, C.G., The history of Parkinson's disease: early clinical descriptions and neurological therapies. Cold Spring Harb Perspect Med, 2011. 1(1): p. a008862.

49. Kempster, P.A., B. Hurwitz, and A.J. Lees, A new look at James Parkinson's Essay on the Shaking Palsy. Neurology, 2007. 69(5): p. 482-5.

50. Williams, D.R., James Parkinson's London. Mov Disord, 2007. 22(13): p. 1857-9.

51. Aarsland, D., et al., Depression in Parkinson disease—epidemiology, mechanisms and management. Nat Rev Neurol, 2012. 8(1): p. 35-47.

52. Gallagher, D.A. and A. Schrag, Psychosis, apathy, depression and anxiety in Parkinson's disease. Neurobiol Dis, 2012. 46(3): p. 581-9.

53. Tan, L.C., Mood disorders in Parkinson's disease. Parkinsonism Relat Disord, 2012. 18 Suppl 1: p. S74-6.

54. Aarsland, D., L. Marsh, and A. Schrag, Neuropsychiatric symptoms in Parkinson's disease. Mov Disord, 2009. 24(15): p. 2175-86.

55. Marsh, L., et al., Provisional diagnostic criteria for depression in Parkinson's disease: report of an NINDS/NIMH Work Group. Mov Disord, 2006. 21(2): p. 148-58.

56. Marsh, L., et al., Psychiatric comorbidities in patients with Parkinson disease and psychosis. Neurology, 2004. 63(2): p. 293-300.

57. Pontone, G.M., et al., Prevalence of anxiety disorders and anxiety subtypes in patients with Parkinson's disease. Mov Disord, 2009. 24(9): p. 1333-8.

58. Pontone, G.M., et al., Anxiety and self-perceived health status in Parkinson's disease. Parkinsonism Relat Disord, 2011. 17(4): p. 249-54.

59. Kirsch-Darrow, L., et al., Dissociating apathy and depression in Parkinson disease. Neurology, 2006. 67(1): p. 33-8.

60. Postuma, R.B., et al., Identifying prodromal Parkinson's disease: pre-motor disorders in Parkinson's disease. Mov Disord, 2012. 27(5): p. 617-26.

61. Postuma, R.B., J.F. Gagnon, and J.Y. Montplaisir, REM sleep behavior disorder: from dreams to neurodegeneration. Neurobiol Dis, 2012. 46(3): p. 553-8.

62. Schulte, E.C. and J. Winkelmann, When Parkinson's disease patients go to sleep: specific sleep disturbances related to Parkinson's disease. J Neurol, 2011. 258(Suppl 2): p. S328-35.

63. Suzuki, K., et al., [Sleep disturbances in patients with Parkinson disease]. Brain Nerve, 2012. 64(4): p. 342-55.

64. Barbeau, A., H. Mars, and L. Gillo-Joffroy, Adverse clinical side effects of levodopa therapy. Contemp Neurol Ser, 1971. 8: p. 203-37.

65. Barbeau, A., et al., Levodopa combined with peripheral decarboxylase inhibition in Parkinson's disease. Can Med Assoc J, 1972. 106(11): p. 1169-74.

66. Barbeau, A., Editorial: Long-term assessment of levodopa therapy in Parkinson's disease. Can Med Assoc J, 1975. 112(12): p. 1379-80.

67. Barbeau, A., High-level levodopa therapy in Parkinson's disease: five years later. Trans Am Neurol Assoc, 1974. 99: p. 160-3.

68. Barbeau, A., [The use of levodopa in diseases other than Parkinsonism]. Union Med Can, 1972. 101(5): p. 849-52.

69. Friedman, J.H., Punding on levodopa. Biol Psychiatry, 1994. 36(5): p. 350-1.

70. Fernandez, H.H. and J.H. Friedman, Punding on L-dopa. Mov Disord, 1999. 14(5): p. 836-8.

71. Hammond, C.J., H.H. Fernandez, and M.S. Okun, Reflections: neurology and the humanities. A punder in Catch-22. Neurology, 2009. 72(6): p. 574-5.

72. Heller, J., Catch-22 1961: Simon and Schuster.

73. Giovannoni, G., et al., Hedonistic homeostatic dysregulation in patients with Parkinson's disease on dopamine replacement therapies. J Neurol Neurosurg Psychiatry, 2000. 68(4): p. 423-8.

74. LeWitt, P.A., J. Dubow, and C. Singer, Is levodopa toxic? Insights from a brain bank. Neurology, 2011. 77(15): p. 1414-5.

75. Parkkinen, L., et al., Does levodopa accelerate the pathologic process in Parkinson disease brain? Neurology, 2011. 77(15): p. 1420-6.

76. Fahn, S., et al., Levodopa and the progression of Parkinson's disease. N Engl J Med, 2004. 351(24): p. 2498-508.

77. Okun, M.S., et al., Piloting the NPF data-driven quality improvement initiative. Parkinsonism Relat Disord, 2010. 16(8): p. 517-21.

78. Voon, V. and S.H. Fox, Medication-related impulse control and repetitive behaviors in Parkinson disease. Arch Neurol, 2007. 64(8): p. 1089-96.

79. Voon, V., et al., Impulse control disorders in Parkinson disease: a multicenter case–control study. Ann Neurol, 2011. 69(6): p. 986-96.

80. Weintraub, D., Dopamine and impulse control disorders in Parkinson's disease. Ann Neurol, 2008. 64 Suppl 2: p. S93-100.

81. Weintraub, D., et al., Impulse control disorders in Parkinson disease: a cross-sectional study of 3090 patients. Arch Neurol, 2010. 67(5): p. 589-95.

82. Weintraub, D., et al., Association of dopamine agonist use with impulse control disorders in Parkinson disease. Arch Neurol, 2006. 63(7): p. 969-73.

83. Shapiro, M.A., et al., The four As associated with pathological Parkinson disease gamblers: anxiety, anger, age, and agonists. Neuropsychiatr Dis Treat, 2007. 3(1): p. 161-7.

84. Limotai, N., et al., Addiction-like manifestations and Parkinson's disease: a large single center 9-year experience. Int J Neurosci, 2012. 122(3): p. 145-53.

85. Rabinak, C.A. and M.J. Nirenberg, Dopamine agonist withdrawal syndrome in Parkinson disease. Arch Neurol, 2010. 67(1): p. 58-63.

86. Moum, S.J., et al., Effects of STN and GPi deep brain stimulation on impulse control disorders and dopamine dysregulation syndrome. PLoS One, 2012. 7(1): p. e29768.

87. Lhommee, E., et al., Subthalamic stimulation in Parkinson's disease: restoring the balance of motivated behaviours. Brain, 2012. 135(Pt 5): p. 1463-77.

88. Zigmond, M.J., et al., Neurorestoration by physical exercise: moving forward. Parkinsonism Relat Disord, 2012. 18 Suppl 1: p. S147-50.

89. Smith, A.D. and M.J. Zigmond, Can the brain be protected through exercise? Lessons from an animal model of parkinsonism. Exp Neurol, 2003. 184(1): p. 31-9.

90. Petzinger, G.M., et al., Enhancing neuroplasticity in the basal ganglia: the role of exercise in Parkinson's disease. Mov Disord, 2010. 25 Suppl 1: p. S141-5.

91. Fisher, B., Intervention that challenges the nervous system confronts the challenge of real-world clinical practice. J Neurol Phys Ther, 2011. 35(3): p. 148-9.

92. Corcos, D.M., C.L. Comella, and C.G. Goetz, Tai chi for patients with Parkinson's disease. N Engl J Med, 2012. 366(18): p. 1737-8; author reply 1738.

93. Hass, C.J., et al., Progressive resistance training improves gait initiation in individuals with Parkinson's disease. Gait Posture, 2012. 35(4): p. 669-73.

94. Snijders, A.H., et al., Bicycling breaks the ice for freezers of gait. Mov Disord, 2011. 26(3): p. 367-71.

95. Snijders, A.H., M. van Kesteren, and B.R. Bloem, Cycling is less affected than walking in freezers of gait. J Neurol Neurosurg Psychiatry, 2012. 83(5): p. 575-6.

96. Alberts, J.L., et al., It is not about the bike, it is about the pedaling: forced exercise and Parkinson's disease. Exerc Sport Sci Rev, 2011. 39(4): p. 177-86.

97. Ahlskog, J.E., Does vigorous exercise have a neuroprotective effect in Parkinson disease? Neurology, 2011. 77(3): p. 288-94.

98. Keus, S.H., et al., The ParkinsonNet trial: design and baseline characteristics. Mov Disord, 2010. 25(7): p. 830-7.

99. Keus, S.H., et al., Improving community healthcare for patients with Parkinson's disease: the dutch model. Parkinsons Dis, 2012. 2012: p. 543426.

100. Munneke, M., et al., Efficacy of community-based physiotherapy networks for patients with Parkinson's disease: a cluster-randomised trial. Lancet Neurol, 2010. 9(1): p. 46-54.

101. Nijkrake, M.J., et al., The ParkinsonNet concept: development, implementation and initial experience. Mov Disord, 2010. 25(7): p. 823-9.

102. Aminoff, M.J., et al., Management of the hospitalized patient with Parkinson's disease: current state of the field and need for guidelines. Parkinsonism Relat Disord, 2011. 17(3): p. 139-45.

103. Gerlach, O.H., et al., Deterioration of Parkinson's disease during hospitalization: survey of 684 patients. BMC Neurol, 2012. 12: p. 13.

104. Gerlach, O.H., V.J. Rouvroije, and W.E. Weber, Parkinson's disease and hospitalization: the need for guidelines. Parkinsonism Relat Disord, 2011. 17(6): p. 498.

105. Chou, K.L., et al., Hospitalization in Parkinson disease: a survey of National Parkinson Foundation Centers. Parkinsonism Relat Disord, 2011. 17(6): p. 440-5.

106. Wexler, A., Mapping Fate: A Memoir of Family, Risk, and Genetic Research1996: University of California Press.

107. Tanner, C.M., et al., Rotenone, paraquat, and Parkinson's disease. Environ Health Perspect, 2011. 119(6): p. 866-72.

108. Goldman, S.M., et al., Occupation and parkinsonism in three movement disorders clinics. Neurology, 2005. 65(9): p. 1430-5.

109. Goldman, S.M., et al., Solvent exposures and Parkinson disease risk in twins. Ann Neurol, 2012. 71(6): p. 776-84.

110. Hancock, D.B., et al., Pesticide exposure and risk of Parkinson's disease: a family-based case-control study. BMC Neurol, 2008. 8: p. 6.

111. Dick, F.D., et al., Gene-environment interactions in parkinsonism and Parkinson's disease: the Geoparkinson study. Occup Environ Med, 2007. 64(10): p. 673-80.

112. Christine, C.W., et al., Safety and tolerability of putaminal AADC gene therapy for Parkinson disease. Neurology, 2009. 73(20): p. 1662-9.

113. Marks, W.J., Jr., et al., Gene delivery of AAV2-neurturin for Parkinson's disease: a double-blind, randomised, controlled trial. Lancet Neurol, 2010. 9(12): p. 1164-72.

114. LeWitt, P.A., et al., AAV2-GAD gene therapy for advanced Parkinson's disease: a double-blind, sham-surgery controlled, randomised trial. Lancet Neurol, 2011. 10(4): p. 309-19.

115. Kaplitt, M.G., et al., Safety and tolerability of gene therapy with an adeno-associated virus (AAV) borne GAD gene for Parkinson's disease: an open label, phase I trial. Lancet, 2007. 369(9579): p. 2097-105.

116. Feigin, A., et al., Modulation of metabolic brain networks after subthalamic gene therapy for Parkinson's disease. Proc Natl Acad Sci U S A, 2007. 104(49): p. 19559-64.

117. Mitka, M., Experimental RNA therapy shows promise against Ebola virus in monkey studies. JAMA, 2010. 304(1): p. 31.

118. Geisbert, T.W., et al., Postexposure protection of non-human primates against a lethal Ebola virus challenge with RNA interference: a proof-of-concept study. Lancet, 2010. 375(9729): p. 1896-905.

119. Feldmann, H., Are we any closer to combating Ebola infections? Lancet, 2010. 375(9729): p. 1850-2.

120. Kravitz, A.V., et al., Regulation of parkinsonian motor behaviours by optogenetic control of basal ganglia circuitry. Nature, 2010. 466(7306): p. 622-6.

121. Bass, C.E., et al., Optogenetic control of striatal dopamine release in rats. J Neurochem, 2010. 114(5): p. 1344-52.